Manual of Small Animal
Postoperative Care

Manual of Small Animal Postoperative Care

Robert Taylor, DVM, MS
Alameda East Veterinary Hospital

Robin McGehee, BA, CVT
Alameda East Veterinary Hospital

A Lea & Febiger Book

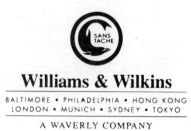

Williams & Wilkins

BALTIMORE • PHILADELPHIA • HONG KONG
LONDON • MUNICH • SYDNEY • TOKYO

A WAVERLY COMPANY

1995

Executive Editor: Carroll Cann
Developmental Editor: Susan Hunsberger
Production Coordinator: Mary Clare Beaulieu
Project Editor: Robert D. Magee

Library of Congress Cataloging-in-Publication Data

Taylor, Robert A. (Robert Augustus), 1946–
    Manual of small animal postoperative care / Robert A. Taylor,
Robin A. McGehee
      p.   cm.
    Includes bibliographical references and index.
    ISBN 0-683-08125-X
    1. Dogs—Surgery—Nursing—Handbooks, manuals, etc.   2. Cats—
of animals—Handbooks, manuals, etc. I. McGehee, Robin A.
II. Title.
SF991.T3   1994
636.089'7919—dc20   94-4929
                                       CIP
                                       Rev.

Copyright © 1995
Williams & Wilkins
Rose Tree Corporate Center
1400 North Providence Rd., Suite 5025
Media, PA 19063-2043 USA

Accurate indications, adverse reactions, and dosage schedules for drugs are provided in this
book, but it is possible they may change. The reader is urged to review the package information
data of the manufacturers of the medications mentioned.

Printed in the United States of America

First Edition 1995

Library of Congress Cataloging in Publication Data

94 95 96 97 98
1 2 3 4 5 6 7 8 9 10

Preface

This manual provides a guideline or frame of reference for veterinary technicians routinely involved in the postoperative recovery of their patients. The first part of the manual develops the principles of postoperative management; the second lists and briefly describes, where necessary, common postoperative problems attendant on the given procedure.

The authors do not intend for this manual to be taken as an absolute; rather, we hope that the guidelines proposed will be taken and modified to fit each clinic or hospital's specific needs and situations. We hope that by providing these guidelines, some degree of standardization will prevail in the profession for the ultimate benefit of our patients.

Contributors

Todd Hammond, DVM
Diplomate, American College Veterinary Ophthalmologists
The Eye Clinic
Golden, Colorado

Janet King, BS, CVT
Bel-Rea Institute of Veterinary Technology
Denver, Colorado

Lisa Lee, BS, CVT*
Bel-Rea Institute of Veterinary Technology
Denver, Colorado

Robin McGehee, BA, CVT
Alameda East Veterinary Hospital
Denver, Colorado

Cynthia Nordberg, DVM
Alameda East Veterinary Hospital

Steven W. Petersen, DVM
Diplomate, American College of Veterinary Surgeons
Denver, Colorado

Douglas R. Santen, DVM
Alameda East Veterinary Hospital
Denver, Colorado

Robert Taylor, DVM, MS
Alameda East Veterinary Hospital, Denver Colorado
Adjunct Associate Professor, Denver University, Denver, Colorado
Clinical Affiliate, Veterinary Teaching Hospital, School of Veterinary Medicine
Colorado State University, Professor, Bel Rea Institute, Denver, Colorado

* Deceased

Contents

I
Guidelines For Postoperative Care

1
General Principles

This manual presents a format for care of the small animal patient in the immediate perioperative period (i.e., 24 hours). Every surgical procedure is unique, and the possible problems and complications that may conceivably develop are endless. In spite of this, most procedures have a small number of common postoperative concerns.

At best, this manual provides standards for patient care and, at the least, stimulates thought and discussion concerning postoperative management.

It is well acknowledged that the surgical patient is subject to life-threatening problems during the immediate postsurgical period, and there are certain principles that can serve as guidelines for those providing postsurgical care.

1. *Recovery period.* The recovery period begins with completion of the operative procedure and cessation of anesthesia, and it continues until the physiologic parameters have normalized.

2. *Pain.* Animals recovering from surgery experience pain. A proactive pain-management protocol should be developed and used for each surgical patient. Using analgesics proactively before the onset of severe pain helps to reduce postsurgical stress and discomfort, and this strategy usually requires less total analgesic drugs.

3. *Monitoring.* Whenever possible, the recovering patient should be continuously observed and key physiologic parameters closely monitored. Ongoing nursing care of the recovering patient is the very basis of the recovery room. Technicians working in the recovery area must be well trained, highly motivated, have good interpersonal communication skills, and work well in stressful situations.

4. *Compassion and concern.* These are expressed by a comforting stroke and a kind word, and they are important aspects of postsurgical nursing care.

5. *Separate area.* Ideally, a separate area of the hospital should be used for the sole purpose of postoperative recovery and be continuously staffed by one or more technicians.

6. *Charting system.* A charting system should be developed so that physiologic trends can be established and observed. Such a system can help to identify potential postsurgical problems, and these trends can then be followed to assess the patient's response to treatment. In addition, careful documentation is a hallmark of good record-keeping. All of the drugs administered, procedures performed, and critical patient events should be charted at the time of administration or occurrence.

7. *Operative team.* The operative team should routinely measure physiologic pa-

rameters during the administration of anesthesia and surgery. These parameters can then be used for comparison during the operative event and recovery. By establishing presurgical patient norms, abnormal parameters are more easily recognized.

8. *Drugs and equipment.* Each hospital recovery area should be equipped with the necessary drugs and equipment to treat postsurgical emergencies and mishaps. The level of equipment and supply inventory can be matched to the level of the surgical procedures performed. For example, chest tubes, chest bottles, and a vacuum system might not be required in the recovery area of a hospital engaged primarily in sterilization procedures.

9. *Training.* Technicians in the recovery area should be well trained in the recognition of life-threatening events and capable of immediate response. In fact, key factors in the successful operation of the recovery area are the training, motivation, and availability of the nursing staff. It is incumbent that the attending veterinarian be summoned or informed immediately so that patient care can be directed. In many universities and large private practices, the recovery area is staffed continuously with both veterinarians and veterinary technicians. In these instances, the veterinarian serves as the director and his or her selection should be based on experience, competence, and or instinct. The director is primarily involved in daily decision-making, directing the administration of medication and levels of physiologic monitoring, and monitoring patient response. Often, the veterinarian assumes direct responsibility for client communication, because life-threatening emergencies frequently occur before or after regular office hours. It is critical that such client communication occur on a timely basis, and only under unusual circumstances should the client not be informed immediately of adverse events. Clients are reassured knowing that their animals are being continuously cared for and that they will be informed ''regardless of the hour'' should an adverse event occur. In many cities, veterinary specialists use day-space in an emergency room; their patients are cared for by the emergency-room veterinarian and staff during the evening.

10. *Mistakes.* Judgment errors and mistakes are inevitable in clinical medicine and surgery. There are no large surveys of veterinary medicine to reflect the number of mistakes made by veterinary personnel. In a recent human study, however, medical house officers made diagnostic mistakes in 33% of cases and reported procedure complications in 11% of patients [1]. We can surmise that equal or greater numbers will occur in veterinary medicine, and it is important to develop constructive mechanisms to deal with this problem. The people involved should meet in private as soon after the mishap as possible to discuss the problem. If the situation is approached in a nonthreatening way, those involved should be able to accept responsibility for their mistakes. Following this constructive dialogue regarding practice modification and procedures, changes can begin. It is vital that all concerned learn from their mistakes and take measures to prevent their recurrence.

REFERENCES

1. Wu AW, et al: Do house officers learn from their mistakes? *JAMA* 265:2089–94, 1991.

2

Postoperative Management

Simply stated, the goal of postoperative care is to insure a safe, normal recovery for the surgical patient. This process should continue until the key physiologic parameters have normalized. The level of postoperative care may be as simple as periodic observation of the patient and recording of temperature, pulse, and respiration, or it may be as complex as continuous, invasive physiologic monitoring.

An awareness of the operative procedure and the common postsurgical problems associated with that procedure can be helpful. Ideally, the level of postsurgical nursing care is matched with the corresponding potential for adverse effects resulting from the procedure or its immediate outcome. Invasively monitoring arterial pressure and pulmonary wedge pressure is not necessary after ovariohysterectomies, whereas simply recording the temperature, pulse, and respiration is not sufficient for monitoring the postoperative progression of a patient recovering from aortic valve replacement. When possible, monitoring of the physiologic systems also is helpful and is covered later in this chapter.

The veterinary surgeon communicates specific postoperative orders and a management plan to the recovery-room staff. It is important to brief the recovery-room staff on the preoperative diagnosis, operative procedure, and predicted outcome. It also is helpful to discuss the most likely postoperative problems and what should be done if they occur. For example, management of a chest tube, presence of multiple intravenous lines, or a closed-wound drainage system all need specific postoperative management plans. It is equally important that a logical plan of action already exists should one of these devices become dislodged or inoperative. The adage "never worry alone" applies here, and an informed staff is better able to prevent problems and also to solve them as they occur. For some routinely performed procedures, uniform postoperative orders can be helpful, because this standardizes the nursing staff's experience with specific medications and procedures. The level of postoperative monitoring is guided by the patient's preoperative status, the operative procedure and its outcome, and the likelihood for significant postoperative problems.

CARDIOPULMONARY SYSTEM

The cardiopulmonary system can be affected profoundly by the surgical procedure itself, anesthetic drugs, and postoperative complications. To monitor and sustain cardiopulmonary function, the following parameters can be used.

5

Temperature, Pulse, and Respiration

Most patients returning from the operating room are hypothermic. Anesthetic drugs block the normal thermoregulatory processes and reduce the metabolic rate. Heat loss through an open chest or abdomen, altered cardiovascular status, and other factors may produce hypothermia. Mild hypothermia is generally well tolerated; however, marked hypothermia can cause a variety of serious complications. Hypothermia causes an increase in the peripheral vascular resistance, decrease in the total-body consumption of oxygen, and a delayed recovery because of reduced biochemical clearance of anesthetic drugs. Marked hypothermia compromises the efficiency of many biochemical functions in the body because of alterations in dissociative constants. In addition, decreases in cardiac contractility, cardiac output, and depressed neurologic status may occur. Marked hypothermia drives the oxygen/hemoglobin dissociation curve to the left (Fig. 2–1), which makes less O_2 available to the tissues.

Smaller patients, because of their greater surface-to-volume ratio, are most susceptible to hypothermia. Reasonable efforts should be made to monitor and maintain euthermia during the operative procedure and recovery period. Core-body temperature can be monitored via an esophageal or rectal probe (Fig. 2–2). Skin temperature correlates well with cardiac output and can be used to monitor the response of the patient. Skin temperature has been used to provide information about peripheral perfusion, because heat is carried to the extremities via blood flow that is in part controlled by the sympathetic venous system. In a normal dog maintained at room temperature (i.e., 68° to 72° C), there is a 3° to 8° C difference between the core-body temperature and toe-web skin temperature [1]. As this difference increases, it indicates reduction of peripheral perfusion, probably associated with vasoconstriction. Toe-web temperature can provide reflections of the cardiac index and peripheral blood flow, and it has been shown to be an inexpensive tool for monitoring animals at risk for developing circulatory shock. A temperature probe can be attached to the ear flap or toe-web skin and be used to monitor the temperature continuously.

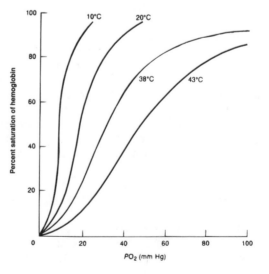

Fig. 2–1. An oxygen hemoglobin dissociation curve showing the relationship between temperature and hemoglobin saturation with O_2 (From Totura G.J., Graloowski S.R.: The Respiratory System. *In* Principles of Anatomy & Physiology, 7th Edn. New York, Harper Collins, 1993).

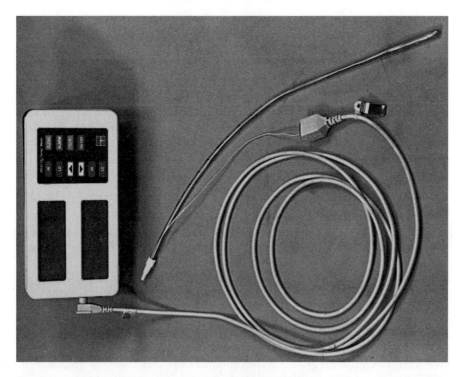

Fig. 2–2. Esophageal stethescope and temperature probe used to monitor core temperature. (Courtesy of David M. Ennis, DVM.)

A relatively new device using infrared thermography also is now available for use in animals. It is designed to evaluate heat radiation from the tympanic membrane. Excellent correlation between the tympanic membrane and core-body temperature has been documented. Although less sophisticated, periodic determination of rectal temperature also can be effective.

Hypothermia is best treated by prevention (Fig. 2–3), but when present, it can be treated with warm blankets (Fig. 2–4), circulating warm water blankets, and massage. Overzealous attempts to reach euthermia by using electric heating pads or hot water bottles often result in severe burns. (Fig. 2–5) The burns from electric heating pads are often extensive and involve the dorsum or lateral aspects of the body. Not uncommonly they are only noticed several days after the incident. These injuries are painful for the patient and create significant tort liability. Studies have shown a great variation in heat production among various brands of electric heating pads [2] that may account in part for the electrical burns. The use of electric heating pads to treat or prevent hypothermia is not recommended.

The occurrence of hyperthermia, while much less frequent, also can be life-threatening. Hyperthermia is occasionally observed in animals anesthetized with ketamine hydrochloride. It seems that the postemergence excitement of the animal results in an elevated core temperature while this is most commonly observed with neuroleptanalgesia, it has been reported with other anesthetic agents as well [3]. This problem

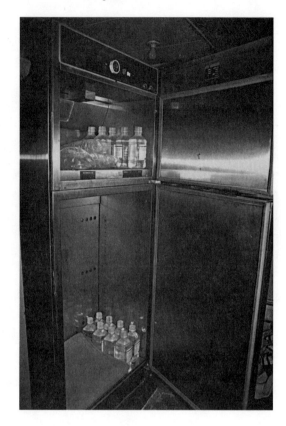

Fig. 2–3. Commercial blanket warmer used to supply warm towels for combating hypothermia. (Courtesy of David M. Ennis, DVM.)

is treated with body-surface cooling (spraying the pads with alcohol); intravenous, intramuscular, or subcutaneous administration of a tranquilizing agent such as acepromazine maleate (0.055 to 0.110 mg/kg body weight); and administering room-temperature intravenous fluids.

Malignant hyperthermia is a genetically determined disorder of muscle metabolism. It has been reported in the dog, pig, and horse, and is discussed in Chapter 8.

The vascular pulse is a compound phenomenon, the result of cardiac output, vascular resistance, blood volume, and neurohormonal control of the cardiovascular system. Monitoring the pulse rate and character is at best an easy but imprecise measure of these parameters. Changes in pulse rate, rhythm, and character can be the harbinger of cardiac arrythmias, infection, blood or fluid loss, and hypoxia. Because redistribution of blood flow often occurs in low-flow sites, it is advisable to check the pulse in several locations. Changes in the rate or character of the pulse should signal the need for more in-depth physiologic monitoring and diagnostic efforts to ascertain the source of the problem. In the dog and the cat, the femoral pulse is the easiest to palpate.

Respiratory rate and volume can be influenced by various drugs, acid–base status, and pain perception. Routinely, this assessment is rudimentary, with only the fre-

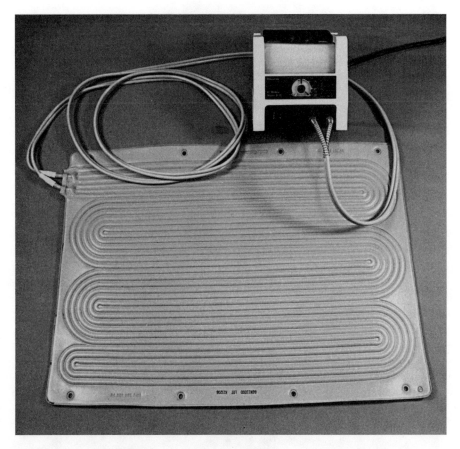

Fig. 2–4. This circulating warm-water blanket can help to prevent hypothermia and is most effective when used in conjunction with anesthesia. (Courtesy of David M. Ennis, DVM.)

quency and character of respiration being recorded. Using a Wright's respirometer (Ferraris Medical Inc. Holland, New York) (Fig. 2–6), one can measure the tidal volume, and values less than 10 mL/kg suggest inadequate ventilation. A gradual increase in the respiratory rate may indicate hypoxemia, secondary pneumonia, acidosis or pulmonary edema. Presurgical assessment of tidal volume, respiratory rate, and acid–base blood gas status is less frequently measured. An additional careful presurgical auscultation can be helpful in detecting the presence of pulmonary edema or pneumonia. When possible, measurement of end-tidal carbon dioxide levels (Fig. 2–7) and evaluation of blood gas values can be helpful in diagnosing and managing problems of diffusion caused by poor respiratory function. Regular auscultation is important to detect any changes in the lungs; fluid rales or an increased harshness in lung sounds can indicate excess pulmonary fluid from overhydration, pulmonary disease, or a failing myocardium. It is difficult at times to differentiate referred upper-airway sounds from fluid rales, but with practice, it can be done.

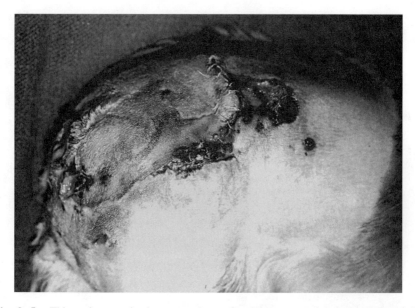

Fig. 2–5. This patient received a severe burn after lying on an electric heating pad for several hours while recovering from anesthesia. (Courtesy of Peter Schwarz, DVM.)

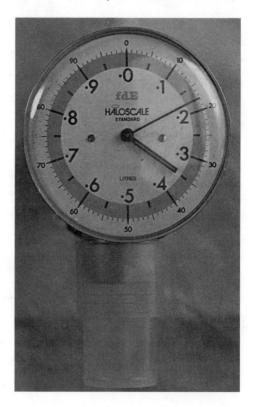

Fig. 2–6. The Wright's respirometer is used to measure tidal volume. Values less than 10 mL/kg body weight suggest hypoventilation. (Courtesy of David M. Ennis, DVM.)

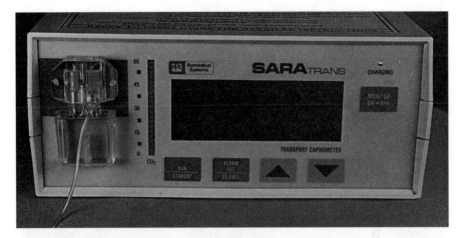

Fig. 2–7. An end-tidal carbon dioxide monitor closely approximates alveolar and pulmonary capillary CO_2 levels and can detect subtle changes in the CO_2 levels. (Courtesy of David M. Ennis, DVM.)

Capillary Refill Time

Capillary refill time is a fairly reliable but somewhat imprecise measurement of perfusion. It is subject to many variables, including the circulatory volume, vascular resistance, cardiac status, and peripheral perfusion. When compared with presurgical values, abnormalities in capillary refill time dictate more careful scrutiny of the factors affecting it.

Packed Cell Volume and Total Solids

When compared with presurgical values, measurements of the packed cell volume (PVC) and total solids (TS) can be useful in assessing blood loss, fluid overload, and hypoproteinemia. This is a quick and inexpensive determination and is readily available in most practices (Fig. 2–8). The PCV/TS determination is important in assessing red blood cell–to–plasma ratios. Serial PCV/TS values and other tests can provide a treatment guideline. If a patient has suffered significant, acute blood loss, both the PCV and TS measurements may be only mildly depressed, but when treated with fluid-volume replacement, the PCV will reflect more appropriately the actual loss of red blood cells. Conversely, animals with protein-losing enteropathies may have a high-normal PCV and low TS measurements.

The difference between peripheral and central PCV can be of prognostic value in assessing the patient's response to treatment [4]. The central PCV is approximately 3% less than the peripheral PCV, and greater differences indicate peripheral hyperfusion. The prognosis is less favorable if this difference continues to increase despite aggressive fluid therapy.

Blood Pressure

Systolic blood pressure can be determined noninvasively through use of a sphygmomanometer and a Doppler-generating device (Fig. 2–9). Use of the Doppler

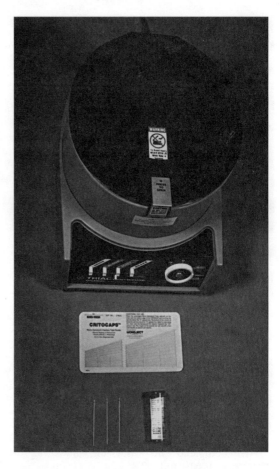

Fig. 2–8. Microhematocrit tube with centrifuge and scale useful in determining packed cell volume and total solids from fresh blood. (Courtesy of David M. Ennis, DVM.)

device creates an audible and easily performed method of monitoring systolic pressure. In operative procedures where invasive monitoring is used, these instruments can be transferred or duplicated in the recovery room and used during the recovery process. The Doppler ultrasonic method of systolic arterial blood pressure measurement is relatively simple and inexpensive. Using a Doppler transducer that detects blood flow and a blood pressure–monitoring cuff enables one to measure indirectly the arterial systolic pressure. In several studies using a Doppler device that measures arterial wall motion, direct systolic pressure was greater than the Doppler systolic pressure [5–8]. A formula using linear notation has been developed for cats and is:

$$DSP + 14 \text{ mm Hg} = FSP,$$

where *DSP* is the Doppler systolic pressure and *FSP* the femoral systolic pressure, both in mm Hg [9,10]. The real value of DSP is to allow frequent blood-pressure measurements to "trend" an animal's clinical course (Table 2–1).

Central venous pressure is the blood pressure in the cranial and caudal (intrathoracic) vena cava. It is influenced by the blood volume, rate of venous return, cardiac function, vascular tone, and thoracic pressure. It is used clinically to monitor the

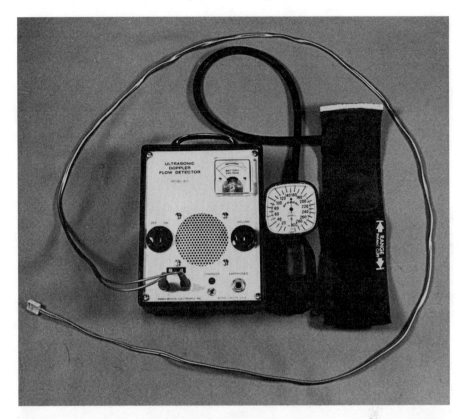

Fig. 2–9. The sphygmomanometer cuff of appropriate size is placed proximal to the Doppler device. As the pressure is slowly released from the cuff, blood begins to flow through the artery, and a Doppler-generated sound is heard. This closely approximates systolic blood pressure. (Courtesy of David M. Ennis, DVM.)

Table 2–1

Summary of Studies Comparing the Doppler Technique of Measuring Systolic Blood Pressure to Directly Measured Systolic Blood Pressure in Dogs and Cats

Author	Animals (n)	Animal Size (kg)	Comparisons (n)	r	Mean Direct Pressure ± sd (mm Hg)	Mean Doppler Pressure ± sd (mm of Hg)	Doppler Adjustment Formula
Freundlich (1972)	12 dogs	10 to 20	480	0.90—0.95	DirP > dsp (Difference up to 30 mm of Hg)	—	Not reported
Garner (1975)	4 dogs	20 to 27	316	0.99	DirP > dsp (Measurement range 50 to 200 mm of Hg)	—	fsp = 0.97 dsp + 3.66 mm of Hg
Weiser (1977)	45 dogs	7 to 36	45	0.93	155 ± 27 (Measurement range 95 to 200 mm of Hg)	155 ± 26	Not reported
Chalifoux (1985)	12 dogs	22.3 (x̄)	72	—	152 ± 36	144 ± 30	Not reported
Klevans (1979)	4 cats	3.5 to 4.0	>16	0.92	DirP > dsp	—	fsp = 1.03 dsp + 7.62 mm of Hg

DirP = direct pressure; dsp = Doppler systolic pressure; fsp = femoral systolic pressure.
From Grandy JL, et al: Elevation of the Doppler ultrasonic method of measuring systolic arterial blood pressure in cats. *Am J Vet Res* 53:1166–1169, 1992.

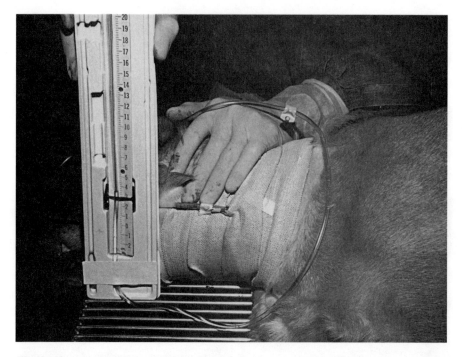

Fig. 2–10. A central venous catheter and manometer can be used to trend fluid-volume replacement in cases of hypovolemic shock and marginal cardiovascular reserves. (Courtesy of David M. Ennis, DVM.)

patient's response to fluid-volume infusion. With normal right cardiac function, central venous pressure is controlled by venous tone and thoracic pressure. Increases in the central venous pressure may indicate volume overload, a change in venous tone, or right cardiac insufficiency. Central venous pressure is monitored by placing a large-size catheter into the cranial vena cava via the jugular vein. The catheter is then connected to a saline-filled water manometer and the central venous pressure expressed in centimeters of saline. The reference point for measure is the right atrium, so in sternally recumbent animals, this corresponds to the manubrium (Fig. 2–10).

Electrocardiograms

In many cases, electrocardiographic (ECG) monitoring is done in the recovery room. Telemetry units (Fig. 2–15) offer ease of use and are recommended for patients after GDV, following cardiac surgery, or in patients with known cardiac disease. The recovery-room staff should be able to detect common arrhythmias such as atrial fibrillation (Fig. 2–11), bradycardia associated with hypokalemia (Fig. 2–12), ventricular tachycardia (Fig. 2–13), and premature ventricular contractions (Fig. 2–14). If significant arrhythmias are detected, a six- or 12-lead ECG should be obtained. While ECGs measure heart rate and allow the detection of arrythmias, the presence of an electrical signal does not in itself guarantee myocardial contractions, nor does it provide information regarding strength of contraction or the cardiac output.

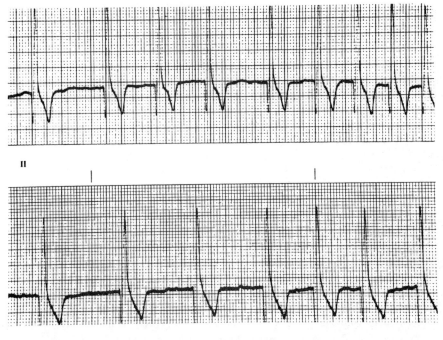

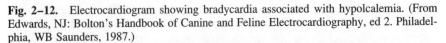

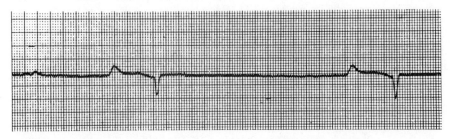

Fig. 2–11. Electrocardiogram showing atrial fibrillation. (From Edwards, NJ: Bolton's Handbook of Canine and Feline Electrocardiography, ed 2. Philadelphia, WB Saunders, 1987.)

Fig. 2–12. Electrocardiogram showing bradycardia associated with hypolcalemia. (From Edwards, NJ: Bolton's Handbook of Canine and Feline Electrocardiography, ed 2. Philadelphia, WB Saunders, 1987.)

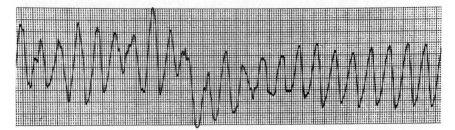

Fig. 2–13. Electrocardiogram showing ventricular tachycardia. (From Edwards, NJ: Bolton's Handbook of Canine and Feline Electrocardiography, ed 2. Philadelphia, WB Saunders, 1987.)

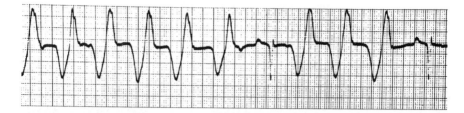

Fig. 2–14. Electrocardiogram showing premature ventricular tachycardia. (From Edwards, NJ: Bolton's Handbook of Canine and Feline Electrocardiography, ed 2. Philadelphia, WB Saunders, 1987.)

Blood Gas and Acid–Base Values

Abnormalities of blood gas and acid–base values are often undiagnosed. Hypoxemia and hypercarbia are frequent postsurgical problems. When possible, evaluation of Po_2, Pco_2, and the arterial or venous pH can be helpful.

The monitoring device for pulse oximetry consists of two light-emitting diodes on one side and a photodetector on the other. It must be placed over a superficial, pulsating arterial bed such as the tail, tongue, pinnae, toe-web, and axillary or inguinal skinfold. The diodes emit two wavelengths that best differentiate between oxyhemoglobin and reduced hemoglobin, and the device is highly accurate in measuring hemoglobin O_2 saturation. Pulse oximetry is much more accurate in measuring hemoglobin O_2 saturation. Pulse oximetry is much more accurate in detecting hemoglobin desaturation than is observation of mucus membrane color, because visual detection of cyanosis is not evident until the hemoglobin saturation falls below 75% (i.e., Pao_2 of approximately 35 mm Hg) [11]. The reliability of pulse oximetry depends on strong arterial pulsation with good light transmission. It is important to select a lightly pigmented area of the skin (or the tongue, which seems the best choice in domestic animals). Hypotension and hypothermia both can alter perfusion and oximetry results; in addition, bright surgical lights and intravenous dyes (Fluorescein) as well as excessive motion can produce artifacts.

Because pulse oximetry provides information about hemoglobin saturation, it is convenient to use the oxyhemoglobin dissociation curve to examine the relationship of O_2 hemoglobin saturation (Sao_2) and the partial pressure of O_2 (Pao_2) (Fig. 2–1). Each 100 mL of oxygenated blood contains approximately 20 mL of O_2, of which 98.5% is transported in chemical combination with hemoglobin. The Pao_2 determines how much O_2 combines with hemoglobin. Note that as the Pao_2 increases from 0 to approximately 50 mm Hg, an almost linear increase occurs in O_2 hemoglobin saturation. After that, the curve becomes much fatter, so that when the Pao_2 is between 60 and 100 mm Hg, hemoglobin is 90% or more saturated with O_2. This means that blood picks up nearly a full load of O_2 from the lungs even when the Pao_2 is as low as 60 mm Hg. Cyanosis occurs when low arterial O_2 saturation forms deoxyhemoglobin, as shown in the following formula:

$$Hb + O_2 \rightleftharpoons HbO_2,$$

where *Hb* is deoxyhemoglobin and *HbO_2* oxyhemoglobin. Cyanosis is evident, because reduced hemoglobin is purple.

The position of the O_2 dissociation curve is shifted by temperature, pH, and $Paco_2$. A rise in temperature, rise in $Paco_2$, or fall in pH shifts the curve to the right. This

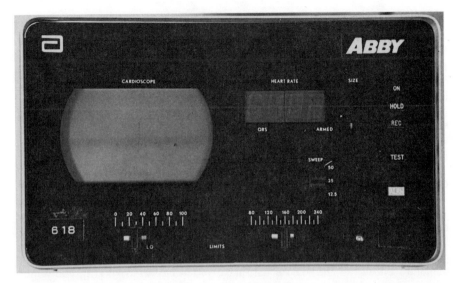

Fig. 2–15. The electrocardiographic telemetry unit can provide continuous electrocardiographic observation and simultaneously minimize patient stress. (Courtesy of David M. Ennis, DVM.)

means that more unloading of O_2 occurs at a given Pao_2. A decrease in temperature, rise in pH, or a fall in $Paco_2$ means that less unloading of O_2 occurs at a given Pao_2.

Pulse oximetry is a simple, noninvasive way to detect unrecognized hypoxemia that might result from hypoventilation or deterioration in alveolar gas exchange. While pulse oximetry is useful for every postoperative recovery, it is very helpful in patients after thoracotomy and those with pre-existing cardiac or pulmonary conditions. The value of pulse-oximetry monitoring is to detect physiologic trends. Oximetry provides assessment of tissue oxygen delivery. When pulmonary gas exchange is diminished, it causes a decrease in O_2 saturation, and in this way, levels of tissue oxygenation can be monitored (Fig. 2–16).

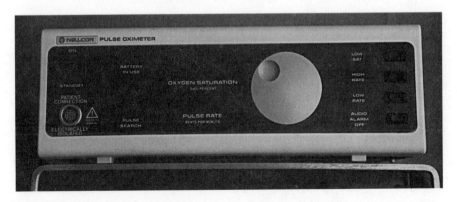

Fig. 2–16. Pulse-oximetry monitoring following anesthesia can quickly rule out hypoxia. (Courtesy of David M. Ennis, DVM.)

Bleeding Disorders

Bleeding disorders can include intraoperative, unreplaced blood loss; ongoing blood loss and coagulation disorders such as von Willebrand's disease; disseminated intravascular coagulation; and thrombocytopenia. In many patients, a presurgical coagulation profile can be helpful. Prompt recognition of inadequate hemostasis because of blood loss or a coagulation disorder can be life-saving. Prolonged oozing or extensive bleeding from a surgical site should be brought to the attention of the surgeon. At this juncture, it is appropriate to expand on von Willebrand's disease, as it is not an uncommon finding and ''is a disease of increasing prominence in the purebred dog population'' [12].

Von Willebrands disease is caused by a reduction or deficiency in von Willebrand's factor, which is a small, adhesive glycoprotein circulating in plasma that is synthesized principally by vascular endothelial cells in the dog [13]. To date, von Willebrand's disease has been recognized in humans, swine, cats, and dogs. Within the canine population, it has been recognized in 50 different breeds, as well as in mixed breeds, and is prevalent in at least eight pure breeds, including Doberman pinschers, golden retrievers, Scottish terriers, Welsh corgis, Shetland sheepdogs, miniature schnauzers, and both standard and toy Manchester terriers [12]. Von Willebrand's disease does not discriminate between genders, and the severity of clinical signs may range from the individual who is an asymptomatic carrier to the animal who bleeds spontaneously. As Table 2–2 shows, it seems prudent to conduct buccal mucosal bleeding times on all purebred Dobermans before surgery. Prolonged buccal mucosal bleeding times occur with von Willebrand's disease and thrombocytopenia. Coagulation tests are usually normal, but the levels of *von Willebrand's factor* can be determined by antigenic assay via electroimmunoassay. These values are expressed as percentages, with normal values between 60% and 172% *vWf:Ag*.

Chemical manifestation of bleeding occurs when plasma levels of von Willebrand's factor drop below 30%u/dL. A screening test for von Willebrand's disease based on platelet agglutination within animal plasma is commercially available (American Diagnostics, Greenwich, CT), and these kits are sufficient for assaying

Table 2–2
Breeds with a High Prevalence of von Willebrand's Disease

Breed	Prevalence (%)
Doberman pinscher	61
Standard Manchester terrier	46
Pembroke Welsh corgi	30
Miniature schnauzer	19
Scottish terrier	16
Toy Manchester terrier	11
Golden retriever	9
Shetland Sheepdog	—*

From Dodds W: Genetic screening for hereditary breeding disorders. *Kal Kan Forum* 1:52–58. 1982
* Insufficient database for reliable estimate.

four samples and are designed for screening "in house." Given the widespread documentation of the disease, however, especially in the dog, it would not be inappropriate to check all surgical candidates for adequate hemostasis before surgery. It behooves all practices involved in surgery to have access to either fresh or frozen plasma, or cryoprecipitate, should a transfusion either during or after the operation be required.

Pretreating all known carriers of von Willebrand's disease before surgery with desmopressin should also be considered (see Chapter 10) [14]. Desmopressin acetate given at 1 μg/kg subcutaneously increases the concentration of von Willebrand's factor for approximately 3 hours. This drug is best given before surgery, and if the procedure lasts longer than 3 hours, it may need to be readministered. Desmopressin acetate has been shown to increase levels of von Willebrand's factor by 150% to 200% following administration [15,16], and the human intranasal preparation has been safely administered subcutaneously in the dog. Plasma cryoprecipitate is rich in coagulation factors, and by nature of the dehydration process, it delivers large amounts of coagulation factors in a small volume. It is administered through an administration set with a 150-μm filter at a dose of 1 bag of cryoprecipitate per 10 kg of body weight 30 minutes before surgery.

CENTRAL NERVOUS SYSTEM

Because most forms of anesthesia temporarily impair functions of the central nervous system, eventual recovery of the animal is predicated on recovery of the central nervous system (see Chapter 8).

Level of Consciousness

As the patient progresses through the planes of anesthetic recovery, there should be a gradual return of the animal's presurgical sensibilities. Abnormalities in this process include coma, seizures, and the exhibition of personality traits unusual for the individual (e.g., lethargy, aggression). The standard is based on how the patient presented presurgically. As the animal regains consciousness, the recovery of key reflexes such as swallowing and blinking are anxiously awaited (see Chapter 8).

Neurologic Status

During the recovery process, the patient's neurologic status should be determined. For example, a patient that was tetraparetic presurgically but becomes tetraplegic during the recovery process indicates progression of the neurologic disease or injury.

Seizures may occur postanesthetically either because of the drugs administered or as a sequelae to the surgical procedure. Ketamine, tiletamide, althesin, methohexitate, and etomidate are the anesthetic drugs most commonly associated with seizures. Metrizamide, a water-soluble myelographic contrast media, may produce seizures in 50% of cases following myelography [17]. Iohexol is a second-generation nonionic contrast medium that is less narcotoxic. A seizure incidence of 10% was reported [18] following iohexol myelography, and male Doberman pinschers seemed to be more sensitive to the drug. Treatment of anesthetic-induced seizures is done with diazepam (Valium) given as an intravenous bolus of 5 to 20 mg and then 0.3 to 0.5 mg/kg/h as a maintenance dose. If metrizamide is the causative agent, bolus administration of glucose or 2.5% glucose in a lactated Ringer's solution may be helpful in controlling the seizure [19].

RENAL FUNCTION

Presurgical assessment of renal function should include urinalysis, blood urea nitrogen and creatinine, and assessment of electrolyte values. Continued monitoring of these during the postoperative period can be helpful in the ongoing evolution of renal function. When anticipated, monitoring of urinary output postsurgically can provide early indications of renal failure and allow for its early, aggressive, and often successful treatment [20]. Urinary output can be monitored by placement of a urinary catheter and a closed urine-collection system. In some instances of urinary obstruction or trauma, a tube cystopexy may be useful as a urinary diversion (Fig. 2–17). These tubes must be securely fastened to the patient and the bladder to prevent dislodgment and leakage of urine either into the peritoneal cavity or subcutaneously.

Intravenous fluid needs should be carefully assessed and determined by surgical fluid administration, intraoperative blood loss, and postsurgical losses. Observation of cardiopulmonary values (i.e., blood pressure, central venous pressure, PCV/TS), electrolyte values, and urinary output can be used to assess fluid needs during the recovery period. The ideal route of fluid administration is oral or enteral, because it is the normal physiologic route. Many postoperative patients are either unwilling or unable to take fluids orally, during the immediate postoperative period. This

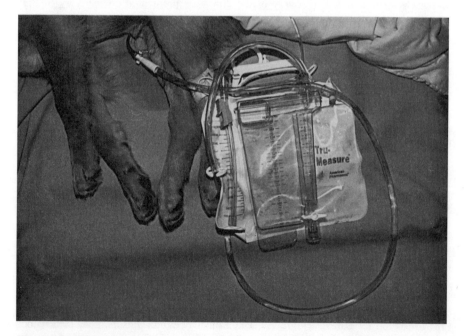

Fig. 2–17. This closed urinary-collection system minimizes urinary infections when catheterization is necessary. It also allows for continuous monitoring of urinary output. (Courtesy of David M. Ennis DVM.)

leaves the option of subcutaneous administration, intravenous catheterization and administration, or intraosseous administration. The subcutaneous route has several disadvantages, the most important being that it is an ineffective way to deliver the large, rapidly perfused amount of fluid sometimes necessary in the postoperative patient.

Intraosseous fluid administration has several advantages, particularly when dealing with neonates or small rodents, inasmuch as intravenous catheterization can prove extremely challenging, especially where shock is present. Catheterization can be achieved by using one or two large-bore needles, and several sites are acceptable, those being the tibia, humerus, and femur [21]. A lesser volume also can be introduced into the iliac crest without deleterious effects. The intraosseous route is acceptable for drug administration as well. Although the administration rate of intraosseous fluid replacement is slightly less than that achieved by the intravenous route, it is nonetheless preferable to have a catheter in place and to initiate fluid-volume replacement rather than to spend precious time searching for a vein.

The rate of administration will vary depending on the route and the needs of each patient. "Gradual intravenous fluid administration to correct dehydration and electrolyte abnormalities is preferred . . . [however] in cases in which hypotensive shock necessitates rapid restoration of circulating volume, faster rates of intravenous fluid administration are required" [21]. Thus, over a 24-hour period where no hypotensive shock is evident, one might use a formula not exceeding 10 mL/kg/h. In case of shock, one would increase the rate to 20 to 30 mL/kg/h. Depending on the number of drops per milliliter delivered by the particular infusion set chosen, one can use the following formula to calculate drops per minute:

$$\text{drops/min} = \frac{\text{drops/mL} \times \text{total volume to be infused (mL)}}{60 \times \text{duration of infusion (h)}}$$

Table 2–3 provides more detail regarding specific caloric and fluid needs based on body weight.

GASTROINTESTINAL FUNCTION

The most common abnormalities of the gastrointestinal system in the recovery period are vomiting, aspiration of saliva, blood in vomitus, and projectile diarrhea. These problems can create devastating complications and require immediate remediation.

HEPATOBILIARY FUNCTION

Hepatobiliary disease can result in coagulation abnormalities. This usually requires some long-standing hepatobiliary disease. An observable sign of hepatobiliary dysfunction is the presence of jaundice, which is best noted by observing discoloration of the sclera. Rarely, however, is the sudden appearance of jaundice observed during the recovery period. Of particular concern regarding hepatobiliary disease in the postoperative patient is insufficient production of clotting factors I, II, V, VII, and X. In addition, the vitamin K–dependent cofactors II, VII, IX, and X may

Table 2–3
Available Fluid Solutions (mEq/L)

	Na	Cl	K	Ca	Mg	Lactate/ Acetate	Osm/L	pH	Cal/L
Plasma (dog)	142	105	4.5	5	2	24	280–300	7.4	3.4
Lactated Ringer's solution	130	109	4	3	0	28	272	6.5	ND
Ringer's solution	147	157	4	5	0	0	314	ND	0
0.85% saline ("normal")	145	145	0	0	0	0	290	ND	0
0.9% saline	154	154	0	0	0	0	308	5.0	0
3% saline	513	513	0	0	0	0	1026	ND	0
0.45% saline in 2.5% dextrose	77	77	0	0	0	0	280	4.5	85
5% dextrose in water	0	0	0	0	0	0	252	4.0	170
10% dextrose in water	0	0	0	0	0	0	505	4.0	340
Lactated Ringer's with 5% dextrose	130	109	4	3	0	28	524	5.0	170
5% dextrose in 0.45% saline	77	77	0	0	0	0	406	4.0	170
Normosol-M	40	40	13	0	3	16	115	ND	ND
Normosol-R	140	98	5	0	3	27 acetate	299	6.2	ND
Normosol-M in 5% dextrose in water	40	40	13	0	3	16	365	5.5	170
50% dextrose	0	0	0	0	0	0	2520		1700
10% mannitol	0	0	0	0	0	0	549	ND	0
15% mannitol	0	0	0	0	0	0	823	ND	0
20% mannitol	0	0	0	0	0	0	1097	ND	0
7.5% $Na HCO_3$	892	0	0	0	0	892 HCO_3	1784	ND	0

ND = not determined.
From Miller, W., et al Conventional and Hypertonic Fluid Therapy: Concepts and Applications In: Murtaugh, R.J., Kaplan, P.M., Veterinary Emergency and Critical Care Medicine, St. Louis, Mosby 1992.

be depleted with hepatobiliary obstruction [22]. Patients with active hepatobiliary dysfunction warrant a presurgical coagulation profile.

REFERENCES

1. Kolata RJ: The Significance of Changes in Toe Web Temperature in Dogs in Circulatory Shock. pg. 21–26, published in "The Proceedings of the 28th Gaines Veterinary Symposium Taskeegee, 1978.
2. Swaim SF, Lee AH, Hughes KS: Heating pads and thermal burning in small animals. *JAAHA* 25:(156–162), 1989].
3. Guze BH, Baster LR: Neuroleptic malignant syndrome. *N Engl J Med* 313:163–165, 1985.
4. Glaff, HI: Standard Technique for the Measurement of Red-Cell and Plasma Volume.

International Council for Standardization in Hematology. (ICSH) Panel on Diagnostic Application of Radioisotopes in Haematology 1973. Vol. 25 p. 801–814.

5. Freundlich JJ, et al: Indirect blood pressure determination by the ultrasonic Doppler technique in dogs. *Curr Ther Res* 14:73–80, 1972.

6. Garner HE, et al: Indirect blood pressure measurement in the dog. *Lab Anim Sci* 25: 197–202, 1975.

7. Weiser MG, et al: Blood pressure measurement in the dog. *J Am Vet Med Assoc* 171: 364–368, 1977.

8. Chalifoux A, et al: Evaluation of the arterial blood pressure of dogs by two noninvasive methods. *Can J Comp Med* 49:419–423, 1985.

9. Klevans LR, et al: Indirect blood pressure determination by Doppler technique in renal hypertensive cats. *Am J Physiol* 237:H720–H723, 1979.

10. Grundy JL, et al: Evaluation of the Doppler ultrasonic method of measuring systolic arterial blood pressure in cats. *Am J Vet Res* pp 53:1166–1169, 1992.

11. Jacobson JD, et al: Evaluation of accuracy of pulse oximetry in dogs. *Am J Vet Res* 53: 537–540, 1992.

12. Hamilton H, Olson P, Jonas L: Von Willebrand's disease manifested by hemorrhage from the reproductive tract: Two case reports. *JAAHA* 21:637–641, 1985.

13. Meyers KM, Wardrop KJ, Meinkoth J: Canine von Willebrand's disease. *Compend Cont Ed Pract Vet* 14:13–22, 1992.

14. Krause JH, et al: Effect of desmopressin acetate on bleeding times and v:Wf in doberman pinscher dogs with von Willebrand's disease. *Vet Surg* 18:103–109, 1989.

15. Johnstone IB, Crane SC: The effects of desmopressin on hemostatic parameters in the normal dog. *Can J Vet Res* 50:265–271, 1986.

16. Johnson GS, et al: DDAVP induced increases in coagulation factor VIII and von Willebrand factor in the plasma of conscious dogs. *J Vet Pharmacol Ther* 9:370–375, 1986.

17. Davis EM, et al: Seizures in dogs following metrizamide myelography. *JAAHA* 17: 642–648, 1981.

18. Lewis DD, Hosgood G: Complications associated with the use of iohexol for myelography of the cervical vertebral column in dogs: 66 cases (1988–1990). *J Am Vet Med Assoc* 200:1381–1384, 1992.

19. Gray PR, et al: Effect of intravenous administration of dextrose or lactated Ringer's solution on seizure development in dogs after cervical myelography with metrizamide. *Am J Vet Res* 48:1600–1608, 1987.

20. Petersen S, Bjorling DE: Surgical techniques for urinary tract diversion and salvage in small animals. *Compendium on Continuing Education.* 12:1699–1709, 1990.

21. Schall W, *General principles of fluid therapy: Symposium on fluid and electrolyte therapy.* Veterinary Clinical Center, College of Veterinary Medicine, Michigan State University.

22. Morrison SA: *Cornell Feline Health Cent Inform Bull* Feline Liver Disease. Cornell Medical College of Veterinary Medicine, Office of Publication Services, Ithaca, NY, No. 8, 1987.

3

Nursing Measures

Nursing care is one of the most important factors in facilitating a smooth, uneventful recovery for the surgical patient. When possible, the recovery area should be staffed with technicians skilled in managing postoperative problems. Often, a kind, soothing hand will settle a "stormy" recovery when all else fails.

FACILITY

When possible, a separate recovery area is desirable. This area should have appropriate supplies of drugs and equipment to handle anticipated problems that are appropriate for the surgical load and level. Often the use of large mats placed on the floor or in cages (Fig. 3–1) can be useful for recovery purposes. The area should be large enough to house the equipment, supplies, and personnel.

When a separate recovery area is unavailable, animals should be recovered in the busiest part of the practice, so they can be continuously observed. Under no circumstances should recovering animals be placed "in the ward" and allowed to recover unattended. All too often, this scenario results in the untimely and unobserved death of the patient. Measures for controlling exhaled anesthetic gas and scavenging are covered in Chapter 8.

PAPERWORK

Although time-consuming, charting the ongoing care of a patient is mandatory. This allows one to discern physiologic trends, manage existing problems, verify current treatment, and recognize emerging problems. Charting also can be very useful in substantiating the level of care in medicolegal questions. A flow chart provides a dynamic document, and such a document can be developed in each practice based on the need and depth of postsurgical monitoring (Fig. 3–2).

PATIENT SUPPORT

When possible, technicians should be responsible for only a small group of recovering patients. Knowing the animal's personality before recovery can be helpful.

24

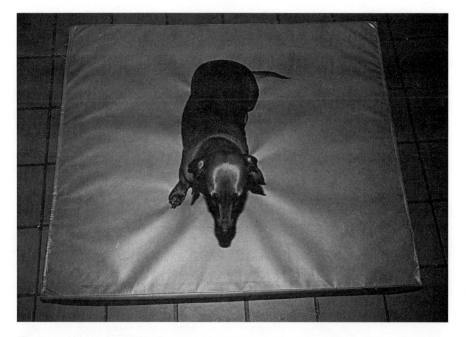

Fig. 3–1. Large, insulated foam pads are placed on the floor for recovering surgical patients. (Courtesy of David M. Ennis, DVM.)

For example, greyhounds fasted before surgery awaken with a voracious appetite, and many animals relax around familiar smells, such as a favorite blanket from home. No degree of sophisticated electronic, physiologic monitoring can supplant the presence of one concerned technician in the recovery room. Given the choice of investing in costly electronic hardware or a recovery-room technician, the latter choice always prevails.

As the animal is presented to the recovery area, it is important that communication occurs to ensure continuity of care. The surgical procedure performed, ongoing medication, intravenous fluid administration, intraoperative problems, and analgesic requirements should be discussed. When possible, this information can be incorporated in the recovery-room charting process (Fig. 3–3). There also are certain specific nursing measures that require attention in the immediate postoperative environment.

Maintenance of Airway and Extubation

Frequently, patients remain intubated when presented to the recovery area. It is important that the tube be kept clear of blood, mucus, saliva, and ingesta (Fig. 3–4). It also is critical to ensure that the tube is not kinked in any way. Extubation is accomplished when the patient begins to cough or buck against the tube; the patient must regain its swallow reflex before extubation. In brachiocephalic breeds, extubation is delayed as long as possible and maintenance of airway patency continuously observed. In this way, soft-palate entrapment, laryngeal edema, and eversion of the lateral ventricles can be prevented.

INTENSIVE CARE UNIT DAILY ORDERS & FLOW SHEET
Alameda East Veterinary Hospital

DATE	ADMISSION DATE	NAME		
WEIGHT TODAY	ADMISSION WEIGHT	CLIENT #		
DR IN CHARGE	HOME PHONE	AGE	BREED	
STUDENT		SEX	CODE	Y ⌐ N ⌐

PROBLEMS

1.
2.
3.
4.

DIAGNOSTICS

1.
2.
3.
4.
5.

COMMENTS

FREQUENCY:		tid bid hid qid					qid		tid
Time:		8:00A	9:00A	10:00A	11:00A	12:00N	1:00P	2:00P	3:00P
TREATMENT:									
1.									
2.									
3.									
4.									
5.									
6.									
7.									
8.									
9.									
10.									
PHYSICAL PARAMETERS:									
Temperature:									
Pulse Rate:									
Respiratory Rate:									
Blood Pressure:									
Mucous Membrane Color: Pink, Pale, Cyanotic, White:									
EKG:									
Attitude:									
Other:									
INTAKE:									
Water:									
Food: (note type and amount)									
Fluids:									
Pump ⌐									
Blood:									
OUTPUT:									
Urine: ⌐ Voided ⌐ Catheter									
Emesis: (record character)									
Diarrhea/Defecation: (record character)									
Other:									
LAB:									
1.									
2.									
3.									
4.									
5.									
6.									
7.									

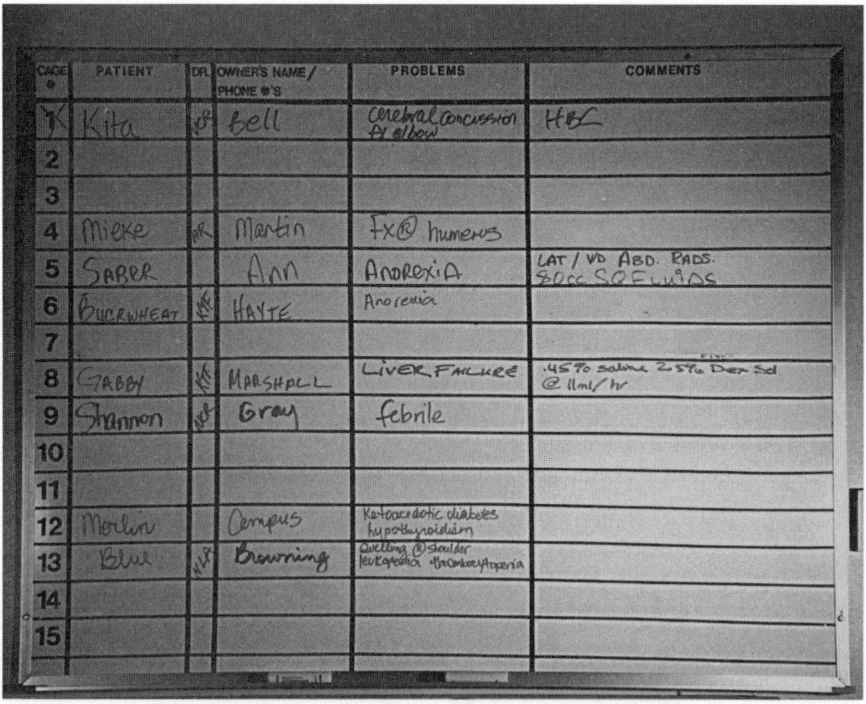

CAGE #	PATIENT	DR.	OWNER'S NAME / PHONE #'S	PROBLEMS	COMMENTS
1	Kita		Bell	cerebral concussion Fx elbow	HBC
2					
3					
4	Mieke		Martin	Fx @ humerus	
5	Saber		Ann	Anorexia	LAT / VD ABD. RADS. 80cc SQ FLUIDS
6	Buckwheat		Hayte	Anorexia	
7					
8	Gabby		Marshall	Liver Failure	.45 % saline 2.5% Dex Sol @ 11ml/hr
9	Shannon		Gray	febrile	
10					
11					
12	Merlin		Campus	Ketoacidotic diabetes hypothyroidism	
13	Blue		Browning	Swelling @ shoulder leukopenia thrombocytopenia	
14					
15					

Fig. 3–3. Recovery-room board to chart all intensive-care-unit patients by procedure, intraoperative complications, monitoring specifics, and serial medications and treatments. (Courtesy of David M. Ennis, DVM.)

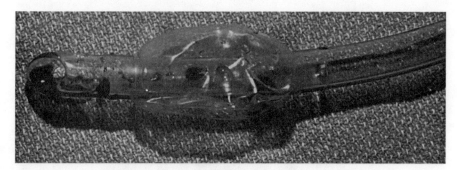

Fig. 3–4. Blood clots in the endotracheal tube may indicate a leaky cuff during oral or laryngeal surgery. Reintubation and suction/lavage of the tracheobronchial tree may be indicated. (Courtesy of David M. Ennis, DVM.)

Control of Body Fluids

Occasional sialorrhea will occur, requiring aspiration of the mouth and airway. If vomiting should occur after extubation, it is important to place the head lower than the chest to encourage gravitational drainage of vomitus and to prevent aspiration. Provisions should be made so that the patient does not become soiled with urine or feces. The use of disposable absorbent pads can enhance patient cleanliness (Fig. 3–5). If urine or fecal soiling occurs, it must be promptly removed; on occasion, the entire perineum must be diligently washed and dried (Fig. 3–6). It may be necessary to clip the hair from the perineum to enhance cleanliness.

Warmth

The patient's core-body temperature should be determined and warm blankets or circulating warm-water devices employed as needed. Most surgical patients will lose 1° to 2° C from body temperature during anesthesia.

Pain Management

A proactive plan of pain control should be developed for each patient. Chapter 6 discusses pain management in greater depth.

Nutrition

In general, early restoration of postsurgical alimentation is encouraged. When to begin is determined by the nature of the presurgical problem and the surgical proce-

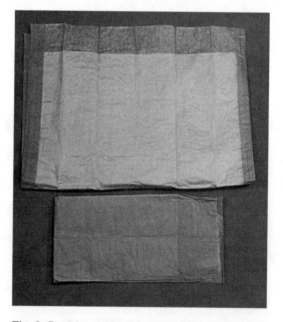

Fig. 3–5. Disposable absorbent pads can be used to absorb urine or feces. (Courtesy of David M. Ennis, DVM.)

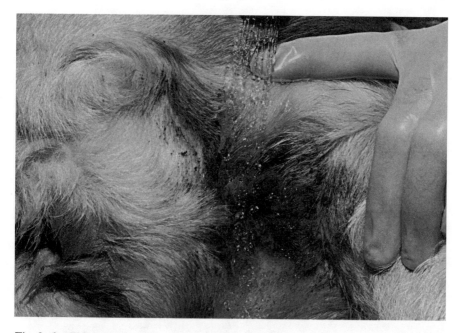

Fig. 3–6. This animal's perineum is being washed and then dried with warm air to remove fecal soiling. (Courtesy of David M. Ennis, DVM.)

dure involved. It is best to discuss alimentation needs with the surgeon. As a rule of thumb, morning surgery means afternoon or evening food, and afternoon or evening surgery means morning food. Beginning 4 to 6 hours postoperatively, small amounts of water are offered. If water is tolerated without nausea or vomiting, small amounts of food and water then can be reoffered frequently thereafter. It is extremely important not to allow overindulgence of water in the immediate postoperative period. This invariably results in vomiting, patient soiling, and discomfort. See Appendix A for more definitive protocols.

Intravenous Catheters

Any patient undergoing general anesthesia should have a vascular access line in place. This may be as simple as a butterfly or as complex as an arterial or venous catheterization, and it is dictated by the complexity of the surgery and the degree of invasive monitoring required (Fig. 3–7 and 3–8). Gaining vascular access during the moribund, hypotensive, postsurgical disaster can be very unrewarding. When extensive postoperative measures are anticipated, more than one vascular access line may be indicated.

Nosocomial Infections

Nosocomial infections are hospital-acquired infections and imply that the patient did not enter the hospital with the infection. Nosocomial infections occur more commonly in university and large referral hospitals. Nosocomial disease is an important postsurgical problem in man, accounting for $1 billion in hospital charges [1]. Nosocomial disease also causes or contributes to patient death in many cases.

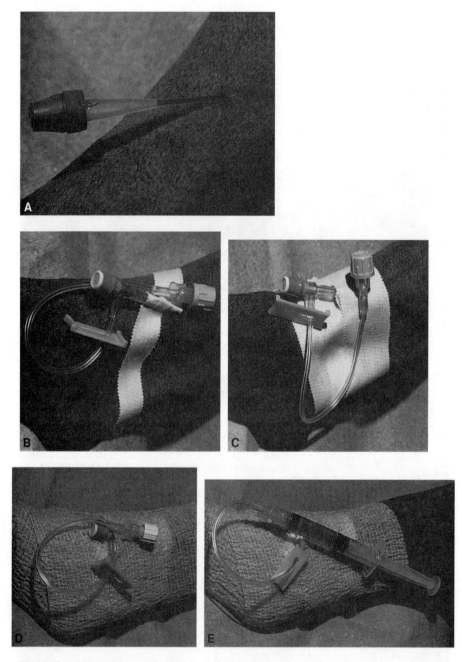

Fig. 3–7. Sequential steps for placing a peripheral catheter. (Courtesy of David M. Ennis, DVM.)

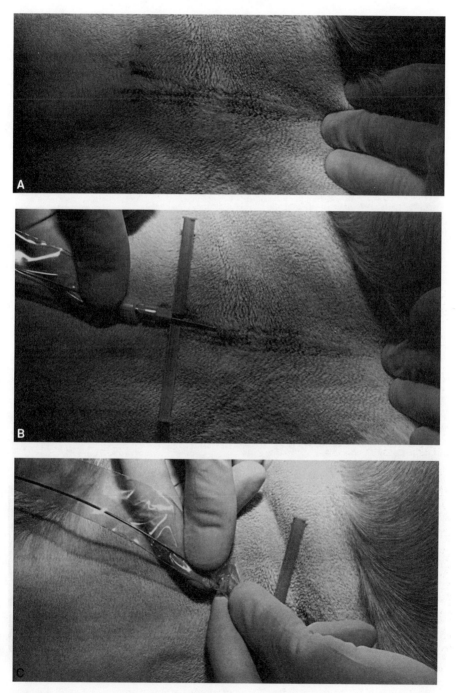

Fig. 3–8. Sequential steps for placing a jugular catheter. (Courtesy of David M. Ennis, DVM.)

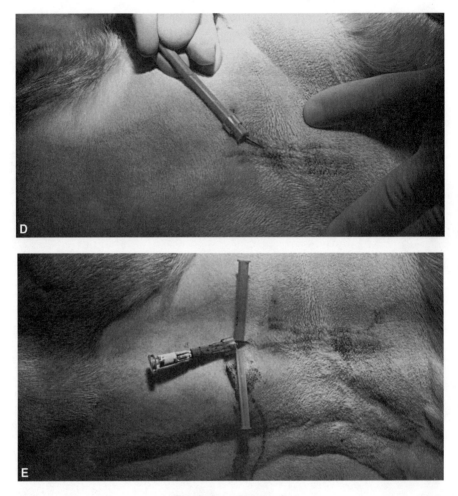

Fig. 3–8. *(Continued)*

Bacteria are the most common veterinary nosocomial infectious agents. Multiple drug-resistant strains of *Escherichia coli, Klebsiella* sp. *Salmonella* sp., and *Pseudomonas* sp. are major nosocomial pathogens [2,3]. The source of bacteria may be the patient's endogenous bacterial flora or exogenous environmental sources. Nosocomial agents are transmitted by direct contact, contaminated equipment, and airborne spread.

Direct contact between patients and the hospital nursing staff is the most prevalent route of infection [3]. There also are a number of recognized predisposing conditions that make a nosocomial infection more likely. The risk of nosocomial disease relates to the presence of an underlying or preexisting disease. Systemic immunosuppressive diseases such as uremia, diabetes, hyperadrenocorticism, neoplasia, and massive trauma predispose the patient to nosocomial disease. Administration of corticosteroids, chemotherapeutic agents, and transfusion may do so as well.

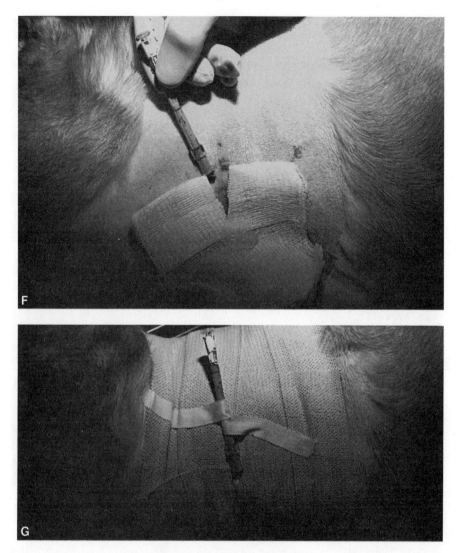

Fig. 3–8. *(Continued)*

Inappropriate use of antibiotics may suppress normal microflora, allowing the colonization of body surfaces by nosocomial bacteria. An understanding of antimicrobial prophylaxis is important to prevent bacterial overgrowth. Oral administration of ampicillin and chloramphenicol and penicillin selectively inhibit intestinal anaerobic organisms and allows the intestinal growth of gram-negative enterics.

The presence of vascular access catheters, urinary catheters, chest tubes, and wound drains are known predisposing factors for nosocomial disease [4]. Catheters that have been pretreated with antiseptics so that the antiseptic bonds to the catheter have been shown to decrease the incidence of disease in rats from catheter-related infections [5]. A biodegradable collagen cuff impregnated with silver salts and placed subcutaneously also has been shown to reduce the incidence of catheter-related infections [6]. While not currently available for use in animals, they undoubtedly will be in the future.

In one veterinary report, infections with *Klebsiella* sp. occurred in 85% of hospitalized patients over a 6-month period [7], whereas 26% of jugular catheters were positive for bacterial growth after being in place for 0.5 to 5.0 days [8]. Following suture stabilization for cranial cruciate rupture, 12 of 66 stifles became infected [9]. In a randomized trial comparing infection rates in ampicillin prophylaxis to those with a placebo in a clean surgery, there was one infection in a patient that had received ampicillin and none in the placebo group. These authors concluded that prophylaxis is not warranted in clean surgical procedures. To minimize and control nosocomial infections, the following guidelines are helpful:

1. Encourage all hospital team members to wash their hands before handling patients, intravenous lines, catheters, drains, and medications.
2. Swab injection ports with alcohol before withdrawing medication.
3. Encourage appropriate use of antibiotics. Try to avoid inappropriate use of prophylactic antibiotics, prolonged use of oral amoxicillin or penicillin, and prophylactic antibiotics when urinary catheterization is anticipated.
4. If possible, wear disposable, sterile gloves when handling catheters and manipulating drains.
5. Clipper blades, electrocardiographic alligator clips, and other routinely used equipment should be cleaned and disinfected between uses.
6. Routinely provide nosocomial surveillance by random culture and susceptibility tests of intravenous and urinary catheters.
7. Intravenous catheters should be covered with a bandage and changed at least every 72 hours.
8. Soiled or moistened bandages should be changed immediately.
9. Minimize handling of fluid-administration sets. When disconnection is necessary, aseptic technique should be used.
10. If indwelling urinary catheters are necessary, they should be connected to closed, sterile collection systems. Routine urinalysis is preferred every 36 hours.
11. All environmental surfaces need prompt and routine cleaning. Try to keep the patient in the same cage throughout its stay in the intensive-care area.
12. Storage containers for swabs, gauze, and so on should be cleaned and sterilized weekly.
13. Recumbent patients should be turned every 2 hours, and coupage can be helpful to minimize retention of pulmonary secretions.
14. When possible, have the same team member treat patients with nosocomial infections, and treat these patients last.
15. Do not share intravenous administration sets or intravenous fluids between patients.
16. Create an awareness of potential risks in your own area, and be willing to comply with recommended procedures designed to minimize nosocomial infections.
17. In large referral hospitals and universities, it may be appropriate to appoint an infection-control committee to develop guidelines for infection prevention, control, and surveillance [3].

REFERENCES

1. Haley RW, et al: The efficiency of infection surveillance and control programs in preventing nosocomial infections in US hospitals. *Am J Epidemiol* 121:182–205, 1985.
2. Lippert AC, Fulton RB, Parr AM: Nosocomial infection surveillance in a small animal intensive care unit. *JAAHA* 24:627–636, 1988.
3. McCurnin DM, Jones RL: Principles of surgical asepsis in *Douglas Slatter,* ed. *Textbook of Small Animal Surgery.* Philadelphia, 1993, WB Saunders, pp. 114–123.
4. Murtaugh RJ: Nosocomial disease. In Murtaugh RJ, Kaplan PM, eds. *Veterinary Emergency and Critical Care Medicine.* St. Louis, Mosby–Year Book, pp. 45–50, 1992.
5. Bach A, et al: Prevention of catheter related infections by antiseptic bonding. *J Surg Res* 55:640–646, 1993.
6. Flowers RH, et al: Efficacy of an attachable subcutaneous cuff for the prevention of intravascular catheter related infection. A randomized controlled trial. *JAMA* 261:878–886, 1989.
7. Glickman LT: Veterinary nosocomial *Klebsiella* infections. *J Am Vet Med Assoc* 179: 1389–1392, 1981.
8. Lippert AC, Fulton RB, Parr AM: Nosocomial infection surveillance in a small animal intensive care unit. *JAAHA* 24:627–636, 1988.
9. Dulisch ML: Suture reaction following extra-articular stifle stabilization in the dog—part II. *JAAHA* 17:572–574, 1981.

4

Postoperative Care of the Wound

Postoperative scrutiny of the wound is important to detect early changes associated with infection, hemorrhage, or dehiscence. Equally important is protecting the wound from external contamination and the animal's tendency to lick, chew, or explore the wound. When possible, the wound should be covered with a sterile dressing. Because the primary function of a surgical dressing is to protect the wound from external contamination, occlusive dressings are preferable. Some surgeons routinely coat the suture line with a topical antibiotic ointment, but it is uncertain whether the beneficial effects of this practice result from the barrier effect of the ointment or the antibiotic. A dressing that becomes saturated with body fluid (i.e., blood, bile, urine) should be changed immediately and the source of the drainage determined. The occlusive bandage can be removed after 48 hours, as studies in animals indicate that the surgical wound is far less susceptible to surface contamination after that time [1]. In general, a support wrap around the injured body part provides comfort to the animal and may relieve some postoperative discomfort.

WOUND CLOSURE

Surgical wounds are closed in three ways. Primary closure implies apposition of the skin edges at the end of the operative procedure with staples, sutures, tape, or glue. Most surgical wounds are closed in this way. Delayed primary closure is used for potentially infected wounds; the wound is left open or reopened until the infection or contamination is controlled and the wound can be closed. Some surgical wounds are intentionally left open and allowed to heal by second intention.

GENERAL PRINCIPLES OF ANTIBIMICROBIAL PROPHYLAXIS

Differentiation between the use of antimicrobial drugs to treat existing infection and to prevent infection must be made. Antimicrobial prophylaxis implies the presence of bacteriocidal levels of antibiotics in the tissue at the time of surgery. This is recommended for procedures with a high risk of infection or in which the presence of infection jeopardizes the success of the procedure or the patient's life. Table 4–1 lists procedures that benefit from prophylaxis.

The timing of antibiotic administration is crucial to success. Bacteriocidal levels

Table 4–1
Surgical Procedures that Benefit from Antimicrobial Prophylaxis

Esophageal resection
Intestinal resection in obstruction
Hernia repair using nonabsorbable mesh
Dental procedures combined with other surgery
Biliary surgery in infection
Perineal hernia repair
Total hip prosthesis
Extensive internal fracture fixation
Pacemaker implantation
Colon resection
Prolonged surgery (>2 h) with extensive tissue manipulation
Lobectomy in infection
Resection of stomach in gastric dilatation volvulus
Resection and reconstruction of the rectum–anus
Open fracture repair
Extensive neurosurgical procedures

(Slatter, D.: Textbook of Small Animal Surgery. Philadelphia, W.B. Saunders, 1993.)

of antibiotics must be in the tissue when the bacteria arrive, and prophylaxis is not effective if the bacteria have been present in the tissue for longer than 3 hours before antibiotic administration. In general, prophylactic antibiotics are given 1 hour before surgery or at the time of intravenous catheter placement immediately before surgery. In many human trials, a single dose of antibiotic has proven to be effective, but usually one or two additional doses are given at appropriate postsurgical intervals to suppress the growth of contaminating organisms [2].

INFECTION

The surgical wound rarely shows signs of acute infection in the recovery ward. Once infected, wounds may show the classic signs of redness, swelling, and drainage 1 to 7 days after the procedure. Infection may occur at any time postoperatively, but the wound is most susceptible during the early postoperative hours (i.e., until an impervious coagulum has formed, sealing the wound). Infections imply the presence of pathogenic microorganisms in the tissue and can result from operative contamination, hematogenous relocation, or postoperative contamination. In general, patients with infected wounds have an elevated body temperature, leukocytosis with a left shift, extraordinary pain, and redness and swelling associated with the incision accompanied by wound drainage.

Whenever possible, laboratory analysis of the fluid and wound aspirates should be performed. A simple Gram stain of the material obtained often can provide immediate information regarding the wound (Fig. 4–1 and 4–2). Microscopes and supplies for performing this quick and simple test should be readily accessible. In addition, the material can be Wright's stained and cultured for both aerobic and anaerobic

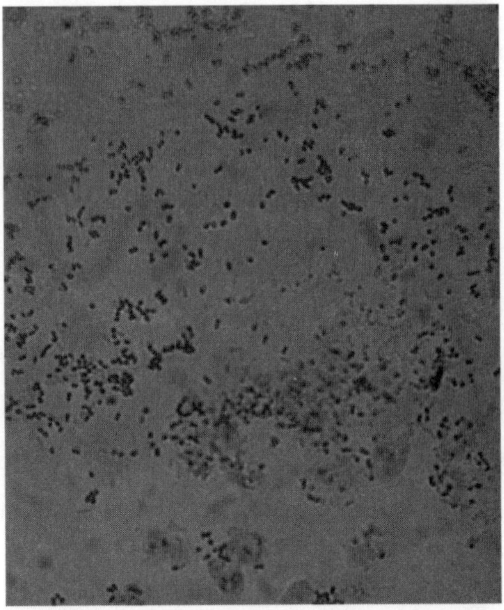

Fig. 4–1. This Gram's stained wound fluid showing numerous gram-positive and gram-negative organisms. (Courtesy of Amy Sorbie, CVT, Alameda East Veterinary Hosp.)

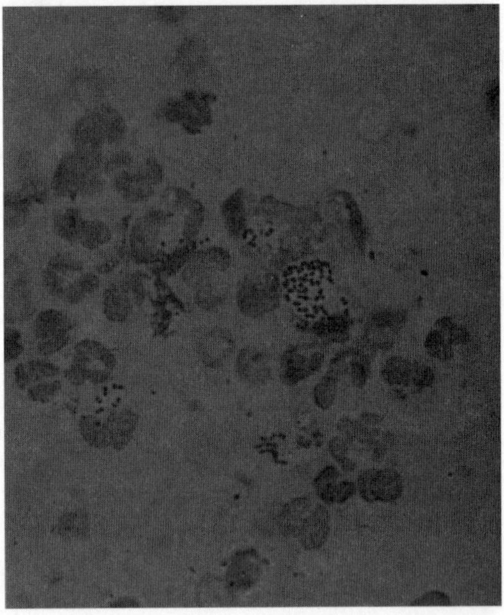

Fig. 4–2. Wright's stained wound fluid illustrating bacteria-laden neutrophils. This is a reliable sign of sepsis. (Courtesy of Amy Sorbie, CVT, Alameda East Veterinary Hospital.)

organisms. Wright's stain can detect the presence of bacteria and help to establish their presence inside or outside of neutrophils. The presence of bacteria-laden neutrophils indicates a wound infection. Postsurgical infections are most commonly caused by staphylococcus, *Escherichia coli,* streptococcus, and pasturella. Of more recent concern is the presence of anaerobic infection. Such infections are characterized by

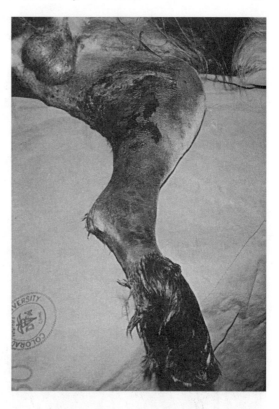

Fig. 4–3. Clear line of demarcation showing the advance of clostridial gangrene on this patient's leg. (Courtesy of David M. Ennis, DVM.)

a foul odor, local pain, and often crepitus. Systemic signs of tachycardia and fever also may be present. Wounds infected by anaerobic organisms require prompt and aggressive debridement, delayed closure, and administration of a broad-spectrum, antimicrobial drug (Fig. 4–3). When a wound is infected, it is important to open the wound to allow adequate drainage. Subsequently, the wound is debrided and subjected to delayed primary closure. The decision to reclose the wound is made based on the animal's clinical progress and evaluation of serial studies of wound fluid as well as Gram and Wright's stained material.

The quantitative determination of bacterial numbers per gram of tissue can be an objective means of determining the timing for wound closure. In general, bacterial numbers less than 10^3 per gram of tissue may safely be resutured. The adage "never let the sun set on an abscess" certainly applies to the presence of an infection in a closed surgical incision.

HEMOSTASIS

Recognition of what constitutes adequate internal or external hemostasis is imperative to ensure satisfactory recovery. Failure to recognize the signs of internal hemorrhage with due alacrity will result in the animal's demise. Prolonged or excessive bleeding along an external suture line will not necessarily have the immediately

Table 4–2
Causes of Blood-Loss Anemia in Dogs

Trauma

Coagulopathies
  Congenital
  Acquired (anticoagulants, hepatic disease)

Platelet disorders
  Thrombocytopenia (immune, drugs, rickettsial diseases)
  von Willebrand's disease
  Functional disorders (drugs, dysproteinemias, thrombopathias)

Splenic rupture
  Neoplasia
  Trauma
  Torsion

Gastrointestinal hemorrhage
  Ulceration
  Neoplasia
  Parasites
  Foreign bodies
  Hemostatic disorders

Epistaxis
  Neoplasia
  Infection
  Hemostatic disorders

(From Crystal, M.A., and Cotter, S.M. Acute Hemorrhage: A Hematologic Emergency in Dogs. *Clinical Hematology* 60(14), 1992.)

devastating effects of massive internal hemorrhage, but it nonetheless should not be taken lightly. In general, oozing hemorrhage should coagulate within 5 minutes. Firm, nonfrictional pressure applied to an oozing wound for 5 minutes often will suffice. One should avoid the temptation to continually dab the wound, as this only removes the coagulum. If 5 minutes of digital pressure on the incision fails to stop the hemorrhage, a coagulopathy may exist, and the surgeon should be notified (Table 4–2).

The most recognizable sign of internal hemorrhage is evidence of pale to white mucus membranes. Because this is an indication of peripheral perfusion and influenced by many factors, pale mucus membranes should be considered in that context. Diminished systolic pressure, tachycardia, and evaluation of serial packed-cell-volume/total-solids determinations are more objective measurements of internal blood loss. In postthoracotomy or postlaparotomy cases, excessive blood from chest tubes or drain lines can be used to assess internal hemorrhage. Once the presence of internal hemorrhage has been ascertained, several steps must be taken:

1. Minimize continued losses. The use of abdominal pressure wraps has been shown to diminish internal abdominal bleeding (Fig. 4–4).
2. Stabilize blood pressure. Application of pressure to a limb can help to elevate systemic blood pressure (Fig. 4–5). The administration of lactated Ringer's or a crystalloid solution to increase the circulating fluid volume and maintain plasma osmolality is crucial (lactated Ringer's solution; 10–90 mL/kg body weight/h; dextran, 10–20 mL/kg/d given over 2–4 h or hypertonic saline [7.5%

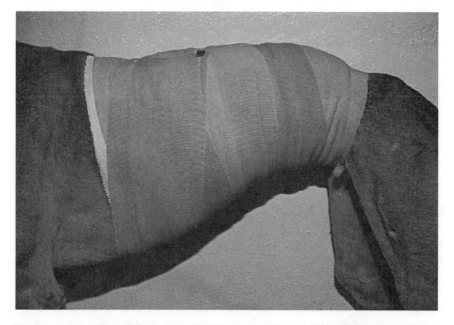

Fig. 4–4. An abdominal belly wrap applies counterpressure to the abdomen. This helps to stop hemorrhage caudal to the diaphragm, increases systolic blood pressure, and facilitates autotransfusion of peritoneal blood. (Courtesy of David M. Ennis, DVM.)

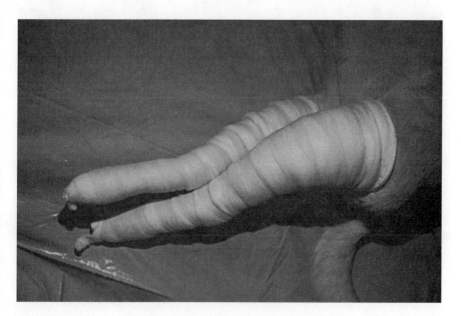

Fig. 4–5. Pressure wraps to the pelvic extremities can provide the same counterpressure as an abdominal belly wrap. (Courtesy of David M. Ennis, DVM.)

solution], 5 mL/kg). Timely evaluation of serial packed-cell-volume/total-solids can help to determine the need for whole blood as opposed to packed red blood cells. One also should consider the use of various vasopressor drugs.

3. Identify and stop the source of hemorrhage. This frequently requires a trip to the operating room and re-exploration of the surgical site. The patient's preoperative status must be optimized before this stressful ordeal.

Hemorrhage associated with a coagulopathy such as von Willebrand's disease, factor deficiency associated with hepatopathy, or a rodenticide-induced coagulopathy can be more insidious. Their detection requires an index of suspicion fortified with coagulation profiles and buccal mucosal bleeding times, ideally beginning presurgically (Table 4–2).

WOUND DISRUPTION

Wound disruption may only involve the superficial layers and usually results from poor technique or judgment error on the part of the surgeon. Failure to drain hematomas, improper application of suture material, and improper wound drainage are all possible causes. When deeper layers are disrupted, there is fluctuant swelling across the wound [3]. The most common sign of abdominal wound dehiscence is serosanguinous discharge from the wound. Wound infection is a factor in 50% of dehiscences [4], and should be ruled out in every case (Fig. 4–6). In abdominal wound dehiscences, peritoneal contents may herniate into the disrupted area. One

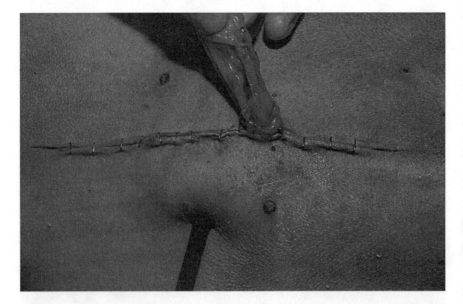

Fig. 4–6. Acute wound dehiscence is noted by soft, fluctuant swelling, often with a small amount of sterile, serosanguinous fluid dripping from the incision when the animal stands. It may be possible to manually reduce the herniated structures into the abdomen. (Courtesy of David M. Ennis, DVM.)

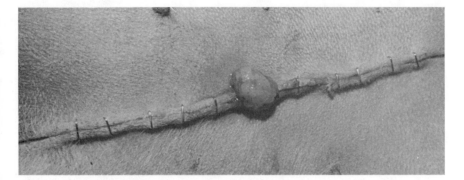

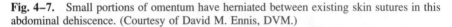

Fig. 4–7. Small portions of omentum have herniated between existing skin sutures in this abdominal dehiscence. (Courtesy of David M. Ennis, DVM.)

may notice small portions of omentum herniating through existing skin sutures (Fig. 4–7), and in severe cases, the animal will remove the skin sutures or staples with subsequent herniation of abdominal contents. Considerable self-mutilation and trauma may occur, to the obvious detriment of the patient. If this occurs, the abdominal contents should be protected with saline-moistened laparotomy pads and a secure belly wrap applied as a temporary measure (Fig. 4–8). The animal's cardiovascular status is stabilized, antimicrobial therapy commenced, and the patient taken to the operating room. There the wound can be debrided, all nonviable tissue removed, and the wound sutured. In severe cases, removal of devitalized intestinal loops and anastomosis must be accomplished.

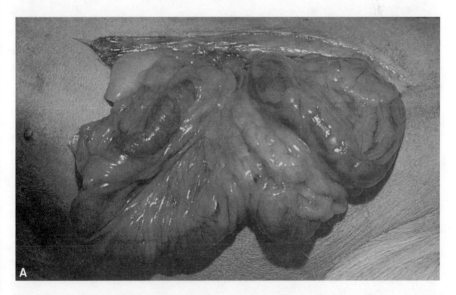

Fig. 4–8. Following abdominal dehiscence, saline-moistened laparotomy sponges are used to protect the abdominal viscera temporarily. This is followed by an abdominal bandage. (Courtesy of David M. Ennis, DVM.)

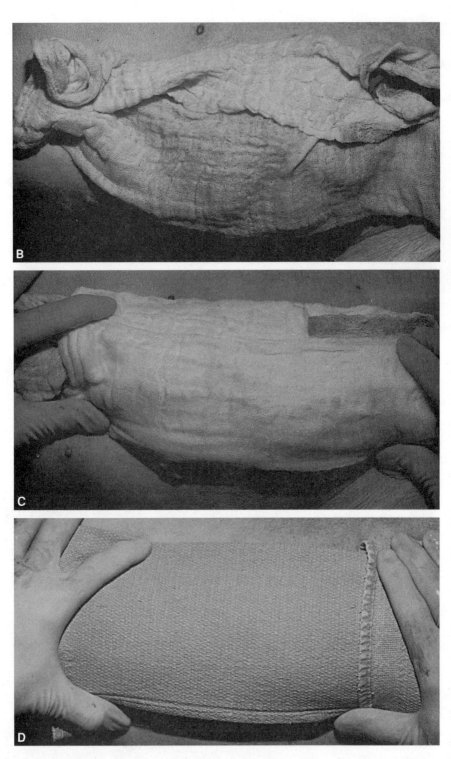

Fig. 4–8. *(Continued)*

HEMATOMAS

The accumulation of large quantities of blood in concert with surgical wounds can pose severe problems. Hematomas provide an ideal inoculum for bacterial growth and delay wound healing. Persistent oozing from the depths of a wound into various tissue planes may produce a hematoma. Wound hematomas must be differentiated from dehiscences, abscesses, and seromas, and needle aspirates of the wound or reexploration with removal of the sutures may be required. Large hematomas must be evacuated, oozing hemorrhage controlled, and the wound packed with sterile packing for delayed primary closure or reclosure.

SEROMAS

A seroma is a delayed wound complication frequently observed from the fifth postoperative day onward. Fluid analysis and needle drainage is recommended initially, but recurrent seromas require placement of a drain (Fig. 4–9). While the presence of a seroma is troublesome, it is seldom life-threatening.

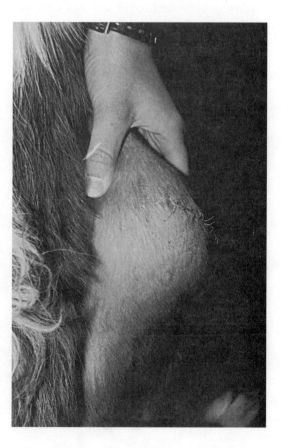

Fig. 4–9. A recurrent seroma following scapulohumeral arthrotomy is drained with a soft rubber tube. (Courtesy of Peter Schwarz, DVM.)

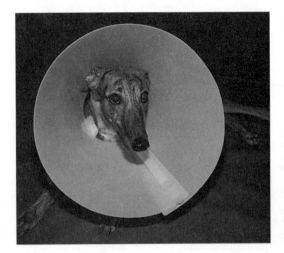

Fig. 4–10. A postsurgical patient fitted with an Elizabethan collar to prevent self-mutilation. (Courtesy of David M. Ennis, DVM.)

WOUND DRAINAGE

Patients suffering from abdominal ascites or pleural or peritoneal effusions may have leakage of these fluids postoperatively. Watertight closure of the primary layers is important. Persistent drainage of pleural or peritoneal fluid delays wound healing and promotes visceral herniation. The defect in the pleura or peritoneum needs accurate closure.

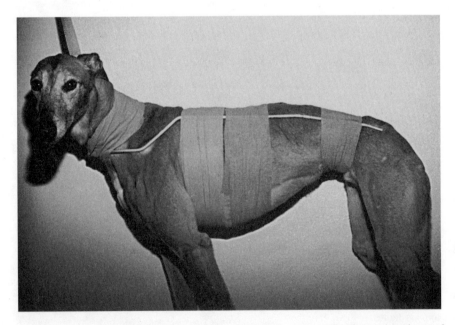

Fig. 4–11. This aluminum side-bar configuration must be custom-fitted to each patient and can be useful in preventing self-mutilation. (Courtesy of David M. Ennis, DVM.)

LICKING

Licking the wound is deleterious and should be prevented at all costs. When in doubt, always assume that the patient will lick and take the appropriate proactive measures. These may include use of an Elizabethan collar (Fig. 4–10), side-bar splints (Fig. 4–11), or appropriate bandaging.

REFERENCES

1. Siemerling GB, Vroman ML: *Infection rate and positive culture rate in 500 consecutive clean sterile surgical procedures in dogs and cats.* 6651-F Backlick Rd., Springfield, Va., Surgical and Orthopedic Service. Unpublished Data.
2. Dipiro JT, et al: Single dose systemic antibiotic prophylaxis of surgical wound infections. *Am J Surg* 152:552–559, 1986.
3. Allen DA, et al: Prevalence of small intestinal dehiscence and associated clinical factors: a retrospective study of 121 dogs. *JAAHA* 28:70–75, 1992.
4. Abernathy CM, Harken AH: *Surgical Secrets.* 2nd Ed. Hanley and Belfus, Inc., Philadelphia, PA, 1991.

5

Postoperative Care of Drains, Tubes, Bandages, and Catheters

Animals often emerge from the operating room with an array of tubes and catheters in place. Proper care of these devices is required to prevent their premature dislodgment, inadvertent contamination, or blockage. In many cases, proper care of these devices is essential for continued life of the patient. For example, ensuring that a chest tube is properly located in the pleural space and is both patent and connected to the proper suction device is crucial for normal respiration. A leaking or improperly positioned chest tube results in an insidious decrease in tidal volume that is often only recognized when the patient is near respiratory failure.

VASCULAR ACCESS CATHETERS

Vascular access catheters range from small butterfly catheters designed for short-term use to elaborate catheters designed for long-term use in a major vessel. In general, any vascular access catheter should be treated with great respect. The proposed area of skin should be clipped and surgically prepared, and once installed, the catheter should be secured to the animal. It also may be advisable to cover the skin entry site with triple-antibiotic ointment.

Butterfly Catheters

Butterfly catheters are designed for short-term use and are valuable for small veins. Their use should be limited to 12 hours. For maximum efficiency, the entire butterfly apparatus should be filled with heparinized saline between fluid or medicinal administrations (Fig. 5–1). Movement of the needle in the vein caused by movement of the patient's extremity frequently damages the vascular intima and accelerates thrombus formation with subsequent venous blockage.

Extended-use Catheters

For longer-term vascular access, placement of a flexible-polypropylene or other synthetic-material catheter is preferred (Fig. 5–2). These may be placed in a peripheral vein, but they are more commonly placed in a major vein (e.g., jugular vein)

48

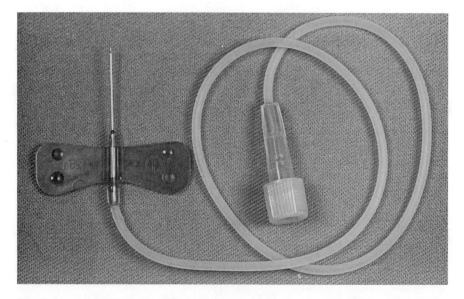

Fig. 5–1. A 26-G butterfly catheter is suitable for small veins. The rigid needle subjects the vein wall to considerable trauma, and the catheter is recommended for short-term (i.e., 12 h) use. (Courtesy of David M. Ennis, DVM.)

or, less commonly, in an artery. As with all intravenous catheters, these must be placed aseptically and treated in an aseptic manner. Ideally, everything that comes in contact with the catheter should be sterile, including sterile gloves worn by the technician when manipulating the catheter apparatus (Fig. 5–3).

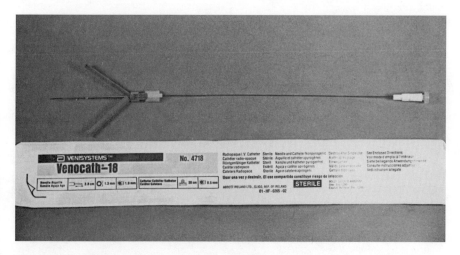

Fig. 5–2. An 18-G jugular catheter can be used for prolonged fluid and maintenance needs. (Courtesy of David M. Ennis, DVM.)

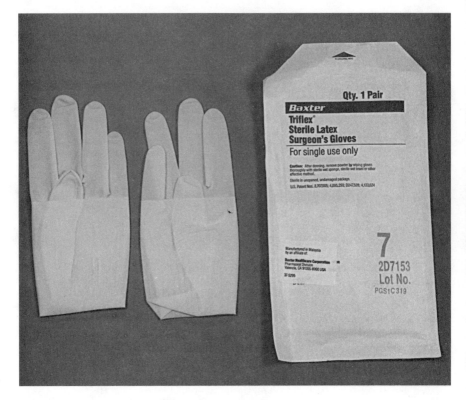

Fig. 5–3. Sterile, disposable gloves are used when the intravenous catheter is manipulated. This is done to minimize the risk of nosocomial infection. (Courtesy of David M. Ennis, DVM.)

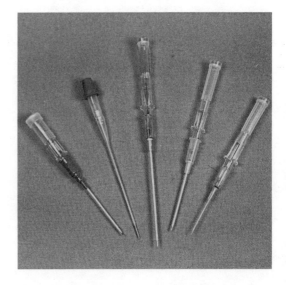

Fig. 5–4. An array of various catheters are available commercially. Pick several that best meet your needs, and use those exclusively. (Courtesy of David M. Ennis, DVM.)

Intermediate-use Catheters

A number of synthetic catheters may be introduced over a needle trocar for placement in a peripheral vein (Fig. 5–4). These catheters may be useful for 24 to 72 hours. They are most commonly used in clinical practice, but one should be cautious about their prolonged use. An inevitable phlebitis results from prolonged catheterization and intravenous administration of fluid. An animal attempting to remove a catheter after 24 to 48 hours probably does so because it hurts.

Catheter Care

To prevent coagulation and thrombus formation, periodic flushing of the catheter with heparinized saline is helpful. The entire catheter apparatus should be bandaged to prevent contamination and to keep the animal from licking it. Indwelling catheters require a great deal of attention, and there is no excuse for an animal to suffer from a severely swollen limb and the consequential pain of fluid extravasation.

Catheters should be removed as soon as they are no longer needed; in some cases, the use of an armboard or splint is necessary to prevent kinking of the proximal vein (Fig. 5–5). With many routine procedures, the catheter is removed once the animal's physiologic variables have normalized and the calculated volume of fluids has been administered. On catheter removal, the wound is compressed and lightly bandaged. A small amount of antibiotic ointment also is placed over the skin wound (Fig. 5–6). Once hemostasis has occurred, this bandage should be removed, and under no circumstances should the animal be released with this bandage in place or the bandage left in place overnight.

Intravenous Catheter Complications

Thrombosis occurs around all indwelling catheters and may occur within 30 minutes of their placement [1]. This often results in thrombophlebitis and is manifested

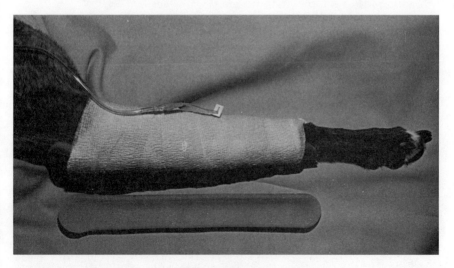

Fig. 5–5. An armboard facilitates fluid administration in this patient and can be fashioned from plastic splint material. (Courtesy of David M. Ennis, DVM.)

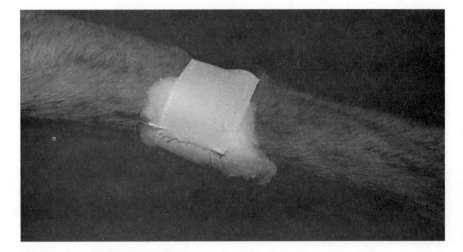

Fig. 5–6. A light bandage and antibiotic ointment are used to cover the catheter site following removal of the device. (Courtesy of David M. Ennis, DVM.)

by local pain, perivascular swelling, and palpation of a cordlike vein proximal to the catheter.

Catheter-related sepsis can occur because of bacterial contamination from the patient, the environment, or the care provider. Topical application of antibiotic creams can limit skin flora growth and may be helpful [2]. Securing the catheter to reduce motion and bandaging the catheter site to prevent licking are recommended.

Recommended Protocol for Intravenous Catheters

The recommended protocol for intravenous catheters is:

1. Surgical preparation of the entry site.
2. Secure the catheter to the skin with tape or sutures.
3. Apply a small amount of triple-antibiotic ointment around the insertion site.
4. Cover the catheter with sterile 4 × 4 and gauze bandage.
5. Have the care provider handle the catheter using disposable sterile gloves.
6. Change the catheter dressing if it becomes soiled.
7. Wipe the catheter junctions with disinfectant before manipulation.
8. Periodically flush the catheter with sterile, heparinized saline.
9. Remove the catheter as soon as it is not needed.
10. Protect the insertion site after catheter removal with antibiotic ointment and a bandage for 2 to 6 hours.

Appropriate Catheter Sizes

The flow rate in milliliters per minute is influenced by the diameter of the intravenous catheter and the height of the fluid container above the patient.

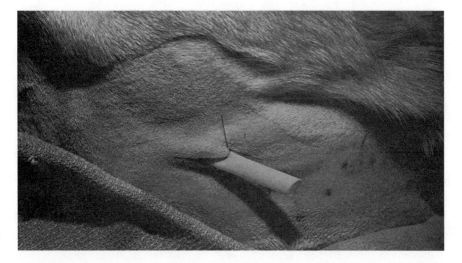

Fig. 5–7. Penrose drain used to allow fluid to drain passively from an abscess. (Courtesy of David M. Ennis, DVM.)

DRAINS AND TUBES

Drains and tubes may allow for passive movement of body fluids externally (Fig. 5–7), be used to instill material into a body cavity (Fig. 5–8), or be used to actively aspirate body fluids. Table 5–1 provides a catheter reference list.

It is important that drains be securely fastened to adjacent tissues to prevent

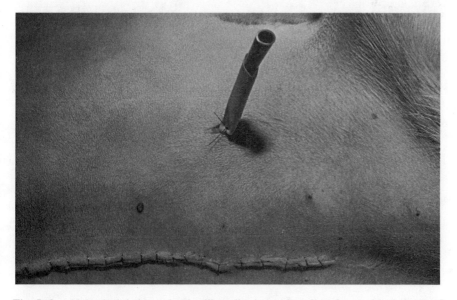

Fig. 5–8. Abdominal drain used to instill medication and to allow for passive drainage of fluid from the peritoneal cavity. (Courtesy of David M. Ennis, DVM.)

Table 5–1
Catheter Reference List

Procedure	Catheter(s)	Company/Address
Pharyngostomy	Silastic tubing	Dow Corning Corp., Midland, MI
	Rubber all-purpose catheter	Davol, Inc., Cranston, RI
Jejunostomy	PE 190 Intramedic polyethylene tubing	Becton, Dickenson & Co., Parsippany, NJ
	Pedi-tube feeding tube (#14-7306)	Biosearch Medical Products Inc., Somerville, NJ
Gastrostomy	Foley catheter	American Latex Corp., Sullivan, IN
	Bard urological catheter	C.R. Bard Co., Murray Hill, NJ
Nasogastric catheterization	Pedi-tube feeding tube (#14-7306)	Biosearch Medical Products Inc., Somerville, NJ
	Sovereign	Monoject Division of Sherwood Medical, St. Louis, MO
Urethral catheterization	Tom cat catheter (Sovereign)	Monoject Division of Sherwood Medical, St. Louis, MO
	Medi-plus tubing	Medi-Plus Laboratories Inc., Division of Avery Corporation., Chicago, IL
Ureteral catheterization	Rusch catheter	Willy Rusch, 7053 Rommelshausen bei Stuttgart, West Germany
	Red rubber (Sovereign)	Monoject Division of Sherwood Medical, St. Louis, MO
Peritoneal dialysis	Lifecath peritoneal implant	Quinton Instrument Co., Seattle, WA
	Purdue column catheter	Physio-Control Corp., Redman, WA
Thoracostomy	Trocar chest tube	Deknatel, Division of Howmedica Inc., Floral Park, NY
	Red rubber catheter (Sovereign)	Monoject Division of Sherwood Medical, St. Louis, MO
Cystostomy	Foley catheter	American Latex Corp., Sullivan, IN
	Bard urological catheter	C.R. Bard Co., Murray Hill, NJ
Nasal sinus irrigation	PE 190 Intramedic polyethylene tubing	Becton, Dickenson & Co., Parsippany, NY
	Pedi-tube feeding tube (#14-7306)	Biosearch Medical Products Inc., Somerville, NJ
Middle-ear irrigation	Silastic tubing	Dow Corning Corp., Midland, MI
	Pedi-tube feeding tube (#14-7306)	Biosearch Medical Products Inc., Somerville, NJ
Closed suction drainage	Hemovac	Snyder Labs, Division of Zimmer, Dover, OH
Nasal insufflation	Infant feeding tube (#3641)	Davol Inc., Cranston, RI
Intravenous catheterization	IV intrafusor	Sorenson Research Company, Salt Lake City, UT
	Brouviac catheter	Davol Inc., Cranston, RI

From Smeak DD: The Chinese finger trap suture technique for fastening tubes and catheters. *JAAHA* 26: 215–218, 1990.

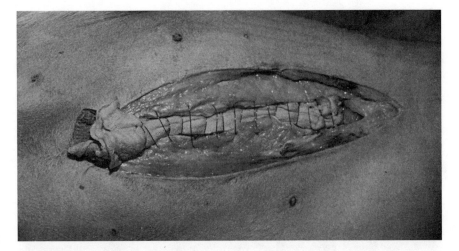

Fig. 5–9. Open peritoneal lavage and drainage used to counteract severe peritonitis. This method of peritoneal lavage is nursing intensive and requires rigorous attention to fluid, electrolyte, and plasma-protein levels. (Courtesy of David M. Ennis, DVM.)

dislodgment and that they be protected from the animal. The chinese finger-trap method is ideally suited for securing many different types of tubes percutaneously. The suture first is loosely anchored to the adjacent skin, then tied to the tubing with a series of surgeon's knots in a criss-crossing pattern to create a friction suture [3]. Drains should be treated as "two-way streets" in that it is possible for contamination to move inward as well as outward. The most common complication of drain use is infection [4]. Drains should be placed and maintained aseptically. If open, the drain should be covered with sterile, absorbent material and changed as often as necessary. The recovery-room team should have a clear understanding of the location and length of time that the drainage device is needed. Close communication with the surgeon regarding this is imperative. In many cases, elaborate peritoneal lavage systems used to combat peritonitis can be challenging to maintain (Fig. 5–9).

Chest Tubes

Placement of a chest tube in the pleural space allows for fluid or air to be evacuated from this space (Fig. 5–10). Dislodgment, leakage, or premature removal of chest tubes can produce life-threatening situations. Several principles must be remembered:

1. To be certain of the tube placement, radiograph the chest to ascertain its placement (Fig. 5–11).
2. Low-level, 2- to 4-cm, water-negative pressure applied intermittently is best for pleural-space evacuation and lung re-expansion.
3. When in doubt, place a chest tube; needle aspiration is useful for diagnosis only.
4. Make sure the tube is clear and patent (Fig. 5–12).

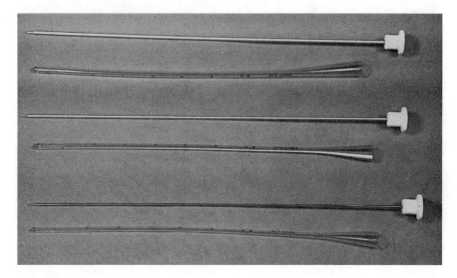

Fig. 5–10. An assortment of chest tubes must be available to match patient size. (Courtesy of David M. Ennis, DVM.)

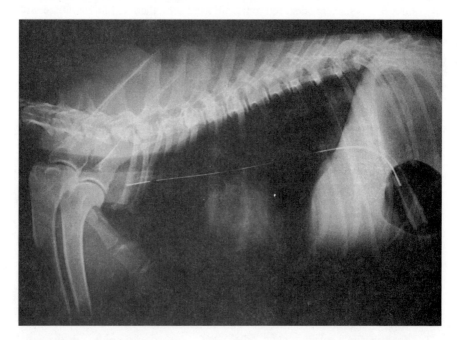

Fig. 5–11. Radiograph showing a chest tube correctly placed in the pleural space.

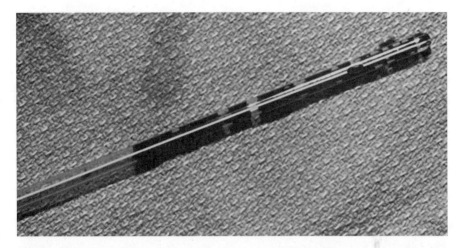

Fig. 5–12. Nonfunctional chest tube filled with coagulated blood. (Courtesy of David M. Ennis, DVM.)

5. When using a fenestrated tube, make sure that all of the holes are within the pleural space and none are in the subcutaneous tissues or distal to the skin incision.
6. The tube must be fixed securely to the skin to avoid dislodgement by the patient's movement (Fig. 5–13).
7. All connections between patient valves or suction devices must be both air- and water-tight and ideally secured with loops of stainless-steel wire (Fig. 5–14).
8. When using chest bottles and a water seal, it is important that the patient be above the water level to avoid gravitation of the water into the pleural space (Fig. 5–15, 5–16).

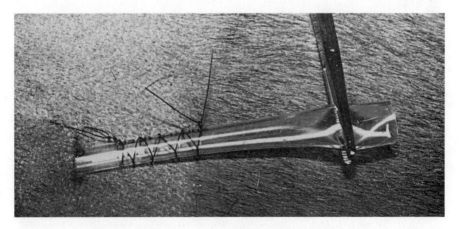

Fig. 5–13. A suggested method for securing a chest tube to the patient. (Courtesy of David M. Ennis, DVM.)

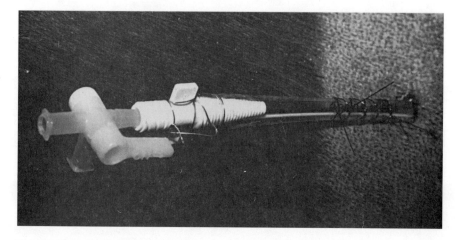

Fig. 5–14.   Stainless-steel suture used to secure all chest-tube fittings. (Courtesy of David M. Ennis, DVM.)

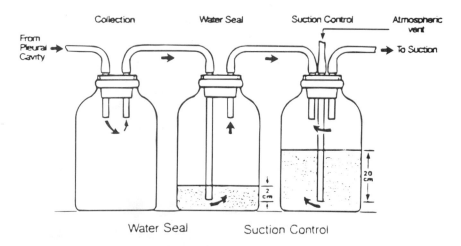

Fig. 5–15.   Three-bottle chest drainage system. (From Abernathy, C.M. and Harken, A.H.: *Surgical Secrets.* 2nd Ed. Hanley & Belfus, Inc. Philadelphia, PA. 1991.)

9. Removal of chest tubes is dictated by the patient's progress. For example, removal after a noneventful thoracotomy might be accomplished in 24 hours; in other cases, the presence of a tube might be quite lengthy.

Peritoneal Drains

Both passive and active peritoneal drainage may be used. Passive peritoneal drainage allows the gravitational flow of fluids. These drains should be covered with

Pneumothorax

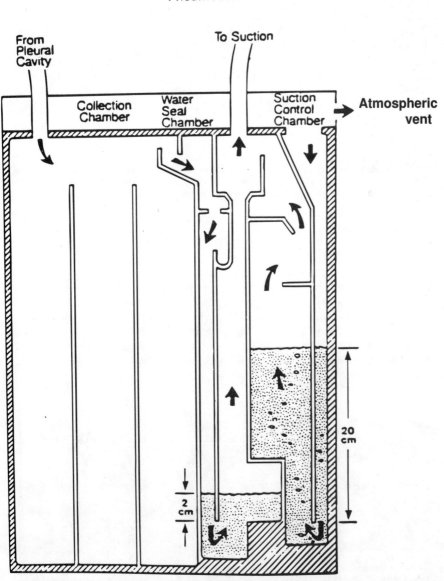

Fig. 5–16.   Another example of a suction device to evacuate air from the pleural cavity. (From Abernathy, C.M. and Harken, A.H.: *Surgical Secrets*. 2nd Ed. Hanley & Belfus, Inc. 1991.)

absorbent material and changed depending on the amount of drainage. Peritoneal drains allowing for infusion and subsequent collection of peritoneal fluid may be treated in a similar manner. In certain severe cases of peritonitis, open peritoneal drainage may be used.

Peritoneal drainage is not a benign procedure. In a study of 12 normal dogs comparing sump drainage (Penrose-Foley catheter along the midline) versus open peritoneal drainage [5], all 12 had mild leukocytosis, hypoproteinemia, peritoneal fluid findings consistent with acute inflammation. Three of the 12 also had positive bacterial cultures at the conclusion of the study. This is a special situation requiring sterile technique, serial anesthesia, and careful bandaging procedures. When this unusual and technically demanding procedure is contemplated, close communication and planning is mandatory.

Wound Drains

Wound drains placed in other areas of the body should be securely fixed to prevent dislodgment. When possible, active suction drains are preferred (Fig. 5–17 and 5–18).

Urinary Catheters

It often is useful to have a urinary catheter present during the operative procedure and recovery period. These catheters must be placed and secured aseptically to adjacent soft-tissue to prevent dislodgment. The catheters also are linked aseptically to a closed urinary collection system. Use of prolonged urinary catheterization invariably leads to urinary tract infection, and catheterization should be confined to the absolute minimum time necessary. Suprapubic catheterization in lieu of uretheral catheterization can be an alternative; the suprapubic catheter may be easier to care for and is well-tolerated [6].

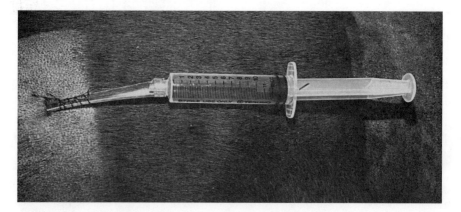

Fig. 5–17. A small hole is drilled in the plunger allowing this syringe to be used as an active wound drain. (Courtesy of David M. Ennis, DVM.)

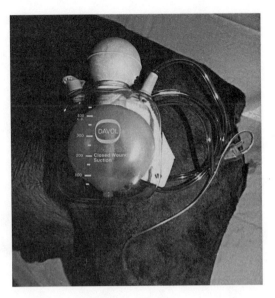

Fig. 5–18. This commercially available, active wound drain must be periodically inspected to ensure that the suction balloon is inflated. (Courtesy of David M. Ennis, DVM.)

SPLINTS, CASTS, BANDAGES, AND FIXATEURS

Soft Bandages

Soft bandages are used to support and protect the wound. It is extremely important that they be kept clean and dry (Fig. 5–19) and that the animal not be allowed to chew or lick them. If the bandage becomes wet or soiled, it must be changed immediately. It is unconscionable that an animal be allowed to wear a urine-soaked bandage. It also

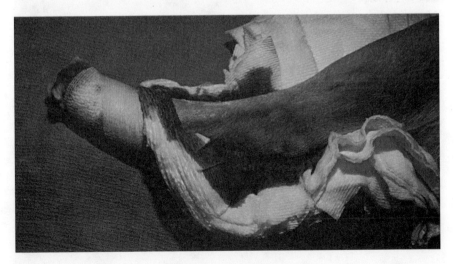

Fig. 5–19. A soiled, urine-soaked bandage may place the animal and success of the procedure at risk. (Courtesy of David M. Ennis, DVM.)

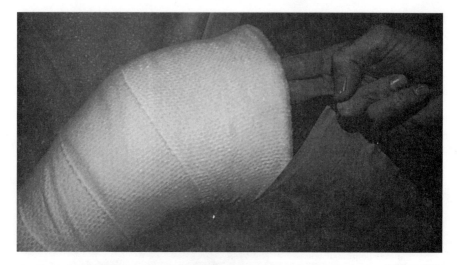

Fig. 5–20. The proximal margin of this bandage accommodates two fingers and is used to check for unneeded tightness. (Courtesy of David M. Ennis, DVM.)

is important that bandages be checked periodically to ensure cleanliness and that they are not too tight. The proximal and distal margins of the bandage should be able to accommodate one or two fingers (Figs. 5–20 and 5–21). This commonly performed procedure has great merit, but if improperly applied or subsequently

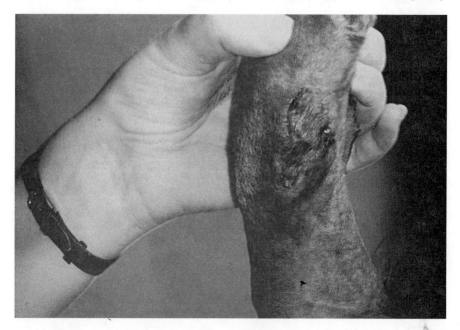

Fig. 5–21. Lower-limb necrosis subsequent to a tight, wet bandage. This limb was subsequently amputated.

neglected, it can cause catastrophic problems. Certain principles of bandaging that provide a guideline for application:

1. When possible, avoid partial-limb bandages. For example, if the elbow needs bandaging, extend the bandage downward to the toes to prevent swelling distal to the bandage.
2. Avoid excessive pressure by using cast padding on the secondary layer, because if the bandage is pulled too tight, this material will give way where other types of padding material may not. Because of its inability to conform to anatomic variations, roll cotton does not evenly distribute pressure. Avoid circumferential pressure caused by bunching of the bandage material, and use extra layers on bony protuberences.
3. Keep the bandage clean and dry. Change soiled bandages immediately.
4. Bandages should provide comfort to the patient. If the animal suddenly begins to lick or actively chew or bite the bandage, the bandage must be removed immediately.
5. Use tape stirrups to stabilize the bandage to the body or extremity (Fig. 5–22).
6. Leave the toes exposed when bandaging extremities, as they serve as a "window" to assess whether adequate blood flow exists distal to the bandage.

Bandages and splints have the following purposes:

1. Protecting the wound.
2. Supporting hard- or soft-tissue repair.
3. Absorbing wound drainage.
4. Enhancing wound healing.
5. Decreasing edema, controlling hemorrhage, and obliterating dead space.

The contact layer used for most surgical wounds is a nonadherent, semiocclusive dressing. Semiocclusive dressings allow the absorption of wound fluids into the intermediate layer of the bandage, but they retain sufficient moisture to prevent dessication of the surgical wound. Examples of nonadherent, semiocclusive contact-layer dressings would be petrolatum-impregnated gauze or the commercially avail-

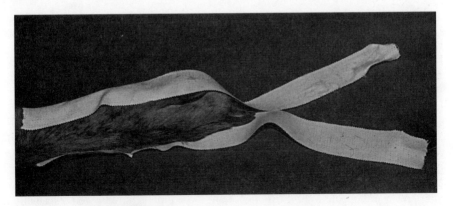

Fig. 5–22. Stirrups placed on an extremity to help stabilize a soft-padded bandage. (Courtesy of David M. Ennis, DVM.)

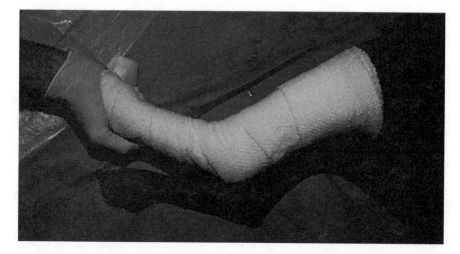

Fig. 5–23. Multiple layers of cast padding are used to protect and support a surgical wound. Usually, two to four layers of cast padding are used. (Courtesy of David M. Ennis, DVM.)

able polyester film–coated cellulose dressing (Telfa Pads, Kendall Co., Boston, Mass.).

The secondary layer is used to pad or support the wound. It also absorbs blood, serum, or wound exudate. This layer can help to obliterate dead space and control edema as well. The material of choice is cast padding, as it conforms to anatomic variables and will give way if pulled too tight. From two to 10 layers may be used depending on the exact need for the bandage (Fig. 5–23).

The tertiary layer consists of surgical tape or elastic tape or wrap, and it secures the other bandage components. This layer may also supply support and desirable pressure to the wound. Ideally, no adhesive material extends proximal to the bandage onto hair coat or the shaved or bare regions of the body.

Splints and Casts

Splints and casts must be kept clean and dry. In general, the same precautions necessary for soft bandages are required when a splint or cast is applied. A broken or missing splint, soiled splint, or a splint that has slipped must be removed and replaced (Fig. 5–24). When in doubt, the surgeon should be consulted before removal of the splint, bandage, or cast.

Splints

Splints may be used for either temporary or adjunctive stabilization of a fracture or injury. In some cases, they may provide the principal stabilization. To be effective, they should span at least one joint proximal and distal to the injury. There are many commercially available splints as well as materials to custom design a splint for an unorthodox orthopedic injury. It is important to pad the extremity well, especially over bony prominences, and fit the splint to the individual patient. For this reason, a customized splint made of fiberglass or casting material is the best choice.

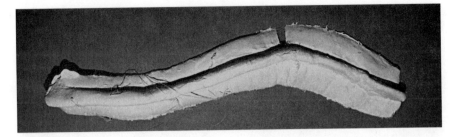

Fig. 5–24. A broken lateral splint needs to be replaced, because stability is compromised. (Courtesy of David M. Ennis, DVM.)

Casts

Casts made of plaster of Paris, fiberglass, or epoxy polymers may be used to:

1. Provide external fixation of appendage fractures.
2. Prevent excessive motion following reconstructive surgery.
3. Provide an adjunct to internal fixation of a fracture.
4. Protect from self-mutilation.
5. Immobilize a limb following surgery.

Because casts usually encircle the limb, great care must be taken in their placement and maintenance.

Casting Procedure

The limb should be clean and dry and any surgical wounds or other injuries covered with a sterile, nonadherent dressing. It is important that the patient is relaxed and the limb cast in a functional, anatomic manner. Tape stirrups are applied on the medial and lateral sides of the foot.

Cast padding (two to three layers) and stockinette are applied to the entire extremity. The plaster casting material or the fiberglass casting tape are applied with an approximately 50% overlap in two layers for small- to medium-sized dogs. In larger dogs, three to four layers may be required.

Casting Concerns

There are a number of concerns regarding casting:

1. Keep the cast clean and dry.
2. Protect the distal aspect of the cast with a walking bar or impervious plastic to prevent wetting when the animal goes outside.
3. Check the animal's toes several times daily for signs of vascular occlusion.
4. Immediately remove the cast if it becomes soiled, wet, has a fetid odor, or the animal begins to chew on it.
5. Casts can be left in place for 2 weeks in a mature animal but should be changed weekly in young, growing animals.

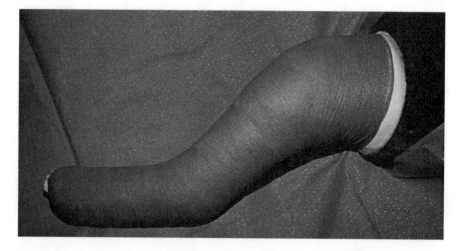

Fig. 5–25.   Application of a pressure wrap (Robert Jones type) to rear leg to support an open tibial fracture. (Courtesy of David M. Ennis, DVM.)

6. Improperly applied or maintained casts can result in devastating pressure sores and result in loss of the limb.

Pressure Bandages

These bandages are used to temporarily support extremity fractures or are applied postoperatively to reduce hemorrhage and edema. Many intermediate layers of cast padding or roll cotton are applied and subsequently compressed with elastic wrap or tape. It is possible to achieve pressure in excess of 50 mm Hg [7] beneath such a bandage, and this pressure exceeds arterial and capillary pressure, causing them to collapse. This type of bandage should in no way be compared with the type of pressure referred to previously for soft-padded bandages. This pressure is intentional and serves a specific purpose, while the other is only detrimental, producing pressure sores because of poor technique. For this reason, caution is advised when applying pressure bandages, and their prolonged application is to be avoided (Fig. 5–25).

External Fixateurs

The use of external fixateurs for fracture repair is common. Protection of the connecting bars and clamps is important to optimize fracture repair. All sharp or protruding points should be covered with soft padding and tape (Fig. 5–26) so that the fixateur does not become ''hung up'' on environmental objects. An Elizabethan collar may be needed to prevent the animal from chewing or licking the fixateur. Skin wounds associated with pin exits should be covered with antibiotic ointment and sterile gauze. Clamp loosening and pin breakage or dislodgment should be brought to the surgeon's attention immediately (Fig. 5–27). Some pin entry/exit wound drainage is to be expected, but excessive hemorrhage or purulent discharge may indicate the presence of active bleeding or infection. Samples of the fluid should be obtained for culture and susceptibility analysis, gram staining, or other diagnostic procedures.

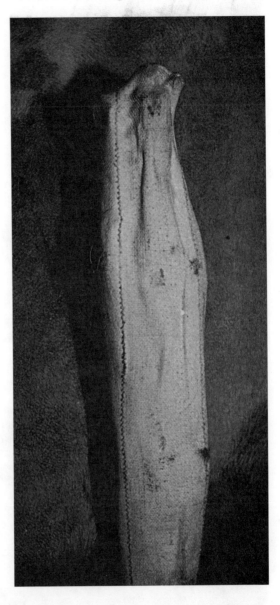

Fig. 5–26. Cotton padding and tape are used to cover and protect the clamps and connecting bars on external fixateurs.

OTHER TYPES OF TUBES

Pharyngostomy Tubes

These tubes must be positioned correctly so that their presence is not uncomfortable, the animal cannot chew the tube, and they can be secured externally to avoid dislodgment (Fig. 5–28). These tubes are usually kept closed, except during use. Incising the neck to allow placement of the tube in the pharynx is done to create

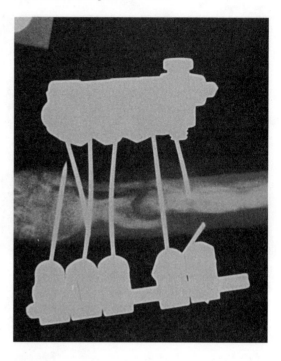

Fig. 5–27. Pin breakage or dislodgment, as in this case, requires immediate attention.

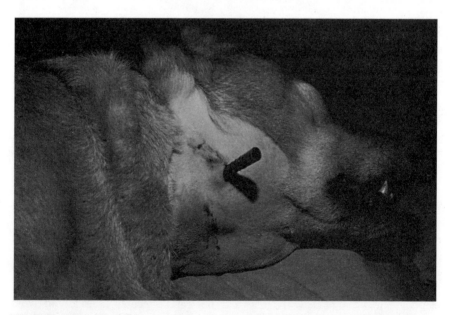

Fig. 5–28. This pharyngostomy tube is ideally positioned and secured with tape and suture to the animal's cervical region. (Courtesy of David M. Ennis, DVM.)

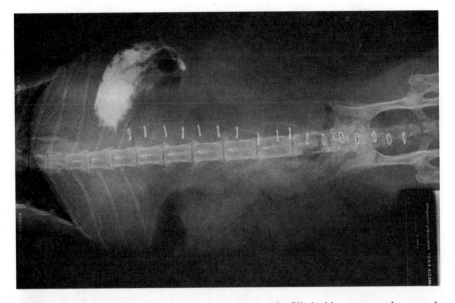

Fig. 5–29. Contrast radiograph showing a gastrotomy tube filled with contrast and accurately positioned in the stomach.

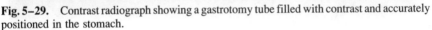

an esophageal feeding tube or bypass the oral cavity with an endotracheal tube. Once the tube has been removed, the pharyngostomy incision is left to heal by granulation. Complications of pharyngostomy tubes include recurrent laryngeal-nerve injury, laryngeal obstruction, coughing, vomiting, aspiration of food, esophagitis, and displacement of the tube.

Gastrotomy Tubes

It is essential that these tubes be placed accurately. When unsure of the location, plain or contrast radiography may be used to ascertain this (Fig. 5–29). Techniques exist for endoscopic-guided gastrotomy-tube placement and allow for accurate, simple placement. Gastrotomy tubes must be secured externally to avoid displacement, because dislodgment may allow peritoneal leakage of gastric contents. The tubes must be placed and secured comfortably for the patient and located so as to be reasonably accessible (Fig. 5–30).

A gastrotomy tube is an excellent method of temporary nutritional support. They are normally placed through a left paracostal laparotomy but can be placed in conjunction with procedures done via a midline laparotomy. Complications associated with a gastrotomy tube include vomiting, peristomal cellulitis, tube removal, and peristomal infection with complication rates as high as 60% [8].

Enterostomy Tubes

Specially designed enterostomy tubes are available (Fig. 5–31) for enteral feeding. Designed for placement in the jejunum, these tubes are constructed and placed so that peristaltic movement does not cause dislodgment. These tubes also must be

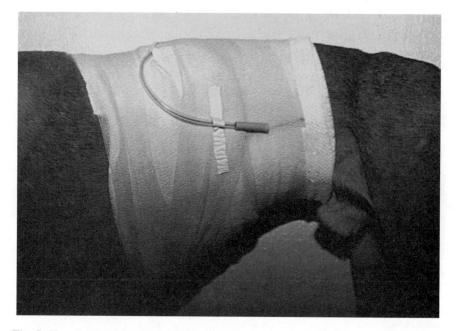

Fig. 5–30. Gastrotomy tube exiting the bandage and accessible for gastric feeding every 4 hours. (Courtesy of David M. Ennis, DVM.)

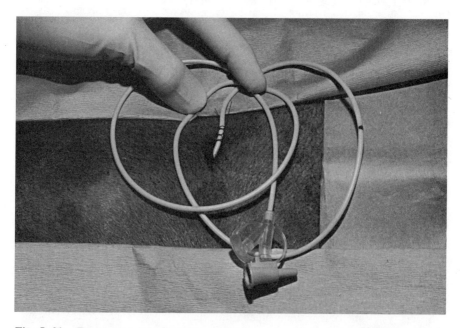

Fig. 5–31. Enterostomy tubes may migrate as a result of intestinal peristalsis, and their small size makes maintenance more demanding. (Courtesy of David M. Ennis, DVM.)

externally secured, protected from the animal, and placed so as to provide easy access. Jejunostomy feeding tubes are indicated when neoplasia, vomiting, regurgitation, or gastroduodenal obstruction prevent feeding from more proximal sites. These tubes may be placed at the time of laparotomy or as a separate procedure. Complications associated with jejunostomy tubes include infection, excessive hemorrhage, leakage of bowel contents, or feeding solutions.

Nasogastric Tubes

Placement of a nasogastric tube may be indicated for gastric evacuation or feeding. Nasoesophageal tubes are preferable, because they do not transverse the gastroesophageal junction. Problems of tube displacement, aspiration of esophageal contents, gastric reflux, and esophagitis may occur; tubes in this location may be poorly tolerated by the animal as well. Careful placement is mandatory, and the tube must be fastened with sutures or cyanoacrylic glue (Fig. 5–32).

Nasal/Oxygen Catheters

Small-diameter nasal/oxygen catheters may be placed postsurgically to provide additional oxygen. In the alert patient, a small amount of topical anesthetic is instilled into the nostril, then an appropriately sized catheter is introduced into the nostril 50% of the length between the nostril and the eye (Fig. 5–33). The catheter is then secured to the nasal region and held with cyanoacrylic cement. When no longer needed, the catheter may be removed using a solvent such as acetone to remove the cement.

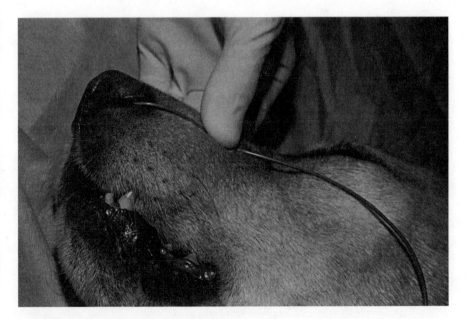

Fig. 5–32.   This nasogastric tube has been secured with cyanoacrylic glue to the nasal region of this patient. (Courtesy of David M. Ennis, DVM.)

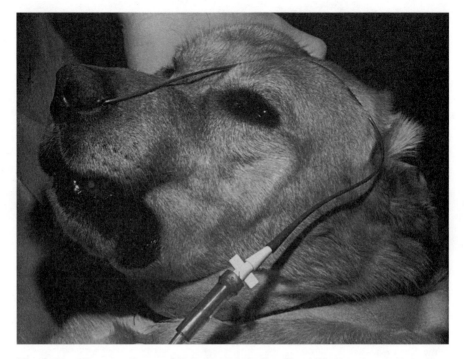

Fig. 5–33. The tube diameter is chosen and the length measured and marked to allow placement of the nasal oxygen catheter. (Courtesy of David M. Ennis, DVM.)

In many postsurgical situations, the best way to administer supplemental oxygen is via a nasal catheter. This avoids the costly and inefficient oxygen cage, and it eliminates forced isolation of the animal. Indications for oxygen therapy include respiratory compromise, altered ventilation/perfusion relationships, circulatory failure, anemic hypoxia, arterial blood values below 60 mm Hg, and other causes of decreased oxygen tissue delivery. Flow rates are to be set at 100 mL/kg body weight.

This procedure usually can be accomplished without sedation or general anesthesia. A small quantity of Cetacaine (Cetylite Industries, Pennsauken, N.J.) is instilled into the nostril. After a short wait, a soft, polyurethane catheter is introduced along the ventral nasal floor and advanced halfway from the nostril to the external end of the nose. The catheter either can be sutured in place or, as we prefer, secured with a small amount of cyanoacrylic cement and then connected to the oxygen transport tubing.

REFERENCES

1. Spurlock SL, Spurlock GH: Risk factors of catheter-related complications. *Compend Cont Ed Pract Vet* 12:241–249, 1990.
2. Norden C: Application of antibiotic ointment to the site of venous catheterization. *J Infect Dis* 120:611–615, 1969.

3. Smeak DD: The chinese finger trap suture technique for fastening tubes and catheters. *JAAHA* 26:215–218, 1990.
4. Cruse, PJE, Foord R: The epidemiology of wound infection: a 10 yr prospective study of 62,939 wounds. *Surg Clin North America* 60:27–40; 1980.
5. Hosgood G, Salisbury SK, DeNicola DB: Open peritoneal drainage versus sump penrose drainage. *JAAHA* 27:115–121, 1991.
6. Dhein CR, Person MW: Prepubic catheterization of 8 dogs with lower urinary tract disorder. *JAAHA* 25:272–276, 1989.
7. Brodell JD, et al: The Robert Jones bandage. *J Bone Joint Surg* 68–13:776–779, 1986.
8. Fulton RB, Dennis JS: Blind percutaneous placement of a gastrotomy tube for nutritional support in dogs and cats. *J Am Vet Med Assoc* 201:697–700, 1992.

6
Management of Postoperative Pain

Surgical procedures and the associated tissue trauma produce various levels of pain in animals. A heightened sense of awareness now exists regarding the pain that animals experience after surgery, and most authorities agree that procedures painful to humans are similarly painful to animals. In the past, veterinarians were reluctant to use analgesia. They felt that some postoperative discomfort kept the animal sedentary and inactive, and they failed to assess adequately pain in animals and were put off by the paperwork required when using narcotics. Veterinarians also failed to recognize signs of pain or discomfort in animals. Pain serves no useful postsurgical purpose, and controlling pain leads to improved surgical recovery.

The Seattle model for pain [1] describes it as a complex phenomenon consisting of four parts: nociception, pain, suffering, and pain behavior. Nociception begins as soon as the stimulus touches the skin through the activation of either alpha, delta, or smaller nonmyelinated C fibers [2]. Nociceptors are particularly numerous in the skin and internal tissue such as the periosteum, joint capsules, arterial walls, muscles, tendons, and membranes of the cranial vault [3]. General anesthetic agents block the brain's response to nociceptive input but not the response of the spinal cord or peripheral nerves, and chemical changes occur there causing the nerves to be hypersensitive to nociceptive input for long periods of time.

Pain is the perception of nociceptive input by the nervous system. Suffering is cerebral response to nociception and often produces personality changes of aggression and alarm. Pain behavior is a complex personality and psychologic response to nociception that occurs primarily in humans.

With this in mind, some general principles of pain control are:

1. Animals experience postsurgical pain, and control of this pain leads to improved surgical recovery (Table 6–1).
2. Proactive pain control is preferable. Agents and dosages for pain control should be discussed as part of the anesthetic protocol and used accordingly. Pain control during surgery decreases the necessary dose of anesthetic drugs as well as reduces postsurgical pain [4].
3. Waiting for the animal to show signs of pain is the least effective method of pain control. Invariably, higher doses of analgesia are necessary at this point, exacerbating the resultant side effects.
4. Proactive nursing care laced with compassion not only hastens recovery but also may decrease the patient's analgesic-medication needs. The patient's envi-

Table 6–1
Expected Postsurgical Pain Response

Surgery	Expected Pain Level
Head, car, throat, dental	Moderate to high
Anorectal	Moderate to high
Ophthalmologic	High
Orthopedic	Moderate to high (upper axial segments, e.g., shoulder/humerus and hip/femur, are very painful)
Amputation	High (transection of large muscle masses and nerves)
Thoracotomy	High (sternal); moderate to high (lateral)
Celiotomy	Mild to high (varies with duration of procedure and procedures associated with major pathologic changes)
Cervical spine	High
Lumbar and thoracic spine	Moderate

From Johnson JM: The veterinarian's responsibility: assessing and managing acute pain in dogs and cats. Part I. *Compend Cont Ed Pract Vet* 13:804–809; Part II. 911–921, 1991.

ronment must be kept clean and dry. It is important to provide adequate padding and to avoid fecal and urinary soiling. When possible, the presence of a loved one during the recovery process can allay the animal's apprehension and ease the recovery.

ANALGESICS

It is beyond the scope of this text to develop a detailed pharmacologic approach to commonly used analgesics. The best method is to select a small group of drugs and methods of administration, know their pharmacodynamics, and use them often.

Opioid Analgesics

These drugs are among the oldest and most widely studied group of analgesics, and they are often used as the standard to which new analgesics are compared. Opioids exert their effect on opioid receptors in the substantia gelatinosa of the spinal cord and the trigeminal nucleus of the brain stem. Five categories of opioid receptors have been described. These account for the varied physiologic responses that occur after administration of various opioid drugs (Table 6–2). Most opioids and their antagonists have different affinities for various receptors. The terms *agonist* (bind and stimulate) and *antagonist* (block and inhibit) have evolved to describe drugs that are competitively antagonistic at one receptor and agonistic at others [5]. The main pharmacologic effect of the opioids is analgesia, while the major disadvantage is generalized depression of the central nervous system. Opioid-produced central nervous system depression precludes their use in some cases of shock, head trauma, and conditions associated with respiratory compromise. They increase intraocular pressure and should not be used in patients with glaucoma or after ophthalmic surgeries. In cats, these drugs may cause dysphoria and psychomotor activity,

Table 6–2
Narcotic Analgesics Used in Dogs

Drug	Potency	Dose	Analgesic Duration (h)	Comments
Morphine	1.0	0.25 to 5.00 mg/kg IM, SQ	4	Respiratory depression, emesis, elevates intracranial pressure, elevates intraocular pressure, metabolized by liver
Meperidine	0.2	2 to 10 mg/kg IM	2	Hypotension with IV injection, painful on injection, metabolized by liver
Oxymorphone	10.0	0.2 mg/kg IM, SQ, IV; do not exceed 60 mg total dose	6	Respiratory depression, auditory hypersensitivity, altered thermoregulation, metabolized by liver
Butorphanol	5.0	0.4 to 0.6 mg/kg IM, SQ, IV	4	Agonist/antagonist, antitussive, antiemetic, ceiling on respiratory depression
Pentazocine	0.3	2 to 3 mg/kg IM	2	Agonist/antagonist, poor analgesic
Fentanyl	100.0	0.04 to 0.08 mg/kg IM, SQ, IV	2	Respiratory depression, auditory sensitization, decreased cardiac output, bradycardia, metabolized by liver
Nalorphine	0.8	11 to 22 mg/kg IM, SQ, IV	2–3	Agonist/antagonist
Naloxone	—	0.04 mg/kg IM, SQ, IV; may be repeated as necessary	2	Pure opiate antagonist; GABA-receptor antagonist

IM = intramuscular; IV = intravenous; SQ = subcutaneous.
With permission from Sackman JE: Pain part II. Control of pain in animals. *Comp Cont Ed Pract Vet* 13:181–193, 1991.

especially if the recommended dose is exceeded. On initial administration, they cause stimulation of gastrointestinal motility, but then subsequently depression, and their use may be contraindicated in patients with gastrointestinal obstruction or intestinal diseases associated with bacteria or toxicosis.

Nonsteroidal Anti-inflammatory Drugs (NSAIDS)

Nonsteroidal anti-inflammatory drugs (NSAIDS) produce analgesia and suppress inflammation by suppressing local prostaglandin production, and they are useful in alleviating low to moderate pain associated with inflammation or prostaglandin production [5]. Inhibition of cyclooxygenase with subsequent decrease in prostaglandin formation produces the analgesic, antipyretic, and anti-inflammatory properties of these drugs. NSAID that have been commonly used in the dog and the cat include aspirin, ibuprofen, flunixin meglumine, naprosyn, phenylbutazone, and meclofenamic acid. These drugs are readily absorbed from the gastrointestinal tract, but there is considerable species variation in hepatic metabolism. NSAID toxicosis is common in dogs and cats [6], with ibuprofen, acetaminophen, aspirin, and endomethicin being the most common causes of toxicosis. The most common signs of toxicosis are vomiting, diarrhea, gastrointestinal bleeding, central nervous system depression, and circulatory disturbances. Ibuprofen has been reported to cause gastric ulceration and perforation in the dog [7]. Doses as small as 8 mg/kg body weight given for 30 days will cause gastric ulceration, and death can occur following one large oral dose. Ibuprofen is not recommended for the dog or the cat [8].

There are a potent group of injectible NSAID currently in use for humans in the United States and for animals in Europe. Ketolorac is an injectible NSAID that has reduced narcotic requirements by 40% in patients recovering from extensive colonic resections [9]. Carprofen and ketoprofen are currently available for animal care in Europe. These drugs inhibit arachadonic acid synthesis by inhibition of the cyclooxygenase cascade and have no central opioid effects. In other human studies, Ketolorac has been shown to be equal to or better than morphine in the treatment of moderate and severe postoperative pain [10]. Ketolorac has been used for analgesia in approximately 100 dogs recovering from major orthopedic surgery at a dose of 0.15 mg/kg given once immediately postoperatively.

ADJUNCTIVE ANALGESICS

Regional Cooling

Regional cooling of the surgical area with circulating-water blankets or cold packs decreases the need for opioid analgesics in humans [11] (Fig. 6–1). Regional cooling with protected ice packs also can be effective, especially after orthopedic procedures on the extremities. We recommend that regional cooling after orthopedic surgeries be used routinely as the patient recovers from anesthesia, then again every 4 to 6

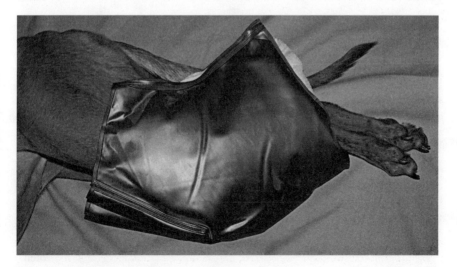

Fig. 6–1. Reusable cold packs for postoperative regional cooling are used routinely after orthopedic surgery. (Courtesy of David M. Ennis, DVM.)

hours for the first 24-hour period postoperatively. Regional cooling reduces the amount of inflammation, allows for early manipulation of the extremity, and helps to alleviate postoperative pain.

Regional Analgesia

In many cases, local nerve blocks after thoracotomy can be helpful in reducing postsurgical pain. Topical anesthetics have been placed in the pleural and peritoneal cavities to reduce pain perception, and in one study, interpleural regional anesthetics provided effective analgesia for 3 to 12 hours [12]. Bupivicaine is better suited for regional analgesia as it has a longer duration of action (i.e., 2–4 hours).

Epidural Analgesia

This is an effective means of providing pain relief lasting from 12 to 24 hours. When opioid agonists are placed in the lumbosacral epidermal space, they rapidly distribute throughout the central nervous system. Epidural anesthesia may be used after laminectomy. The analgesic is placed on the exposed dura before placement of a fat graft and closure.

α-Adrenergic Agonists

Xylazine provides both analgesia and sedation, but adverse cardiovascular side effects often preclude its use after surgery. These include decreased cardiac output and thermoregulation. Tranquilizers alter the animal's response to pain and act as sedarives rather than analgesics. While they lack analgesic properties, they may be combined with analgesics to provide both analgesic and sedating effects.

RECOGNITION OF PAIN

When in doubt, one can assume that if a procedure produces pain or discomfort in humans, it does so in animals as well. As with humans, individual animals react differently to nociception. For example, the field-trial Labrador retriever recovering from cruciate reconstruction may not be as overt in expressing pain as the toy poodle recovering from surgery to correct medial patellar luxation. The following signs are frequently observed when animals are in pain:

Abnormal posture
Aggression
Agitation
Attempts to escape
Changes in personality
Chewing or licking
Failure to groom
Inappetence
Lameness
Pacing
Panting
Salivation

Sinus tachycardia
Tachypnea
Vocalization
Weight loss
Withdrawal

Animals experiencing acute pain often respond by biting or licking the surgical site, while low-grade pain may cause lethargy, inappetence, and behavioral changes. When in doubt, it is better to assume that pain is present and treat it rather than wait for the animal to "show" pain as the result of an arguably painful procedure.

TREATMENT OF PAIN

A pain-awareness protocol should be a part of the presurgical plan. Based on individual preference, availability, and need, a small arsenal of drugs can be chosen

Table 6–3
Nonsteroidal Anti-Inflammatory Drugs Used in Dogs and Cats

Drug	Dose	Frequency (h)	Comments
Dogs			
Aspirin	10 to 25 mg/kg PO	8	Induces gastric ulceration, decreases platelet aggregation
Phenylbutazone	10 to 25 mg/kg PO	8–12	May induce blood dyscrasias, induces gastric ulceration
Dipyrone	25 mg/kg IM, SQ	8–12	Decreases prothrombin, may cause agranulocytosis, causes seizures at high doses
Flunixin	0.5 to 1.0 mg/kg IM, IV	24; 3 dose maximum	Induces gastric ulceration
Naproxen	3 mg/kg PO	24	Induces gastric ulceration
Meclofenamic acid	1.1 mg/kg PO	24	Induces gastric ulceration
Piroxicam	10 mg for dogs under 15 kg PO; 20 mg for dogs over 15 kg PO	24	Induces gastric ulceration
Cats			
Aspirin	10 to 20 mg/kg PO	36–48	Slow metabolism analgesic, antipyretic, decreased platelet aggregation
Phenylbutazone	4 to 5 mg/kg PO	24–36	May cause anorexia, emesis, depression, death
Dipyrone	10 to 25 mg/kg IM, SQ	24	Slow metabolism, good antipyretic

IV = intravenous; PO = orally; SQ = subcutaneous
From Sackman JE: Pain part II. Control of pain in animals. *Comp Cont Ed Pract Vet* 13:181–193, 1991.

and routinely used. The following guidelines might be helpful in choosing an appropriate pharmacy:

1. Animals experience the most severe pain during the first 48 hours after surgery.
2. Opioid agonists given by injection during the procedure or at extubation and during the immediate postsurgical period are appropriate. Parenteral administration, epidural injections, or intravenous infusion also are acceptable methods of administration. Morphine and oxymorphone are readily available, inexpensive, and provide sufficient analgesia (Table 6–2).
3. Opioid agonists–antagonists such as butorphanol, pentazocine, and nalbuphine, while less effective, can be useful when given parenterally for low- to moderate-grade pain.
4. Appropriate use of adjunctive analgesia such as regional nerve blocks, intrapleural regional anesthesia, regional cooling, and tranquilization augment and enhance other types of analgesia.
5. NSAIDs generally are appropriate "go home" medications. They can provide significant analgesia for low-grade pain and can be owner administrated (Table 6–3). As new, patented, injectible NSAIDs become available for use in animals they will have a role in providing analgesia for moderate- to severe-grade pain.
6. Extensive orthopedic procedures, thoracotomies, ocular surgery, and plastic surgical procedures produce significant nociception postoperatively. Diseases such as primary bone tumors, regional ischemia, and pancreatitis are associated with high levels of pain. Certain abdominal procedures such as ovariohysterectomies, cystotomies, and enterotomies seem to be less painful in animals than in humans.

REFERENCES

1. Loeser JD: Perspectives on pain. In Turner P, ed. *Clinical pharmacology and therapeutics.* Baltimore, 1980, University Park Press.
2. Hyman, SE and Cassem NH: *Pain II.* (1983–1994 . . .) Publisher: Carl Peckham Snow, New York, NY. [pgs 1–17] Pain II. (within chapter) Current Topics in Medicine (within) Scientific American Vol. 1. Editor in Chief Edward Rubenstein Editor Daniel D. Federman.
3. Lasagna L: The management of pain. *Drugs* 32(suppl 4):1–7, 1986.
4. Johnson JM: The veterinarian's responsibility: assessing and managing acute pain in dogs and cats—part II. *Compend on Cont Ed* 13:911–921, 1991.
5. Sackman JE: Pain part II, control of pain in animals. *Compend on Cont Ed Pract Vet* 13:181–193, 1991.
6. Hardy E: *ACVS proceedings.* Miami 1992, Published by American College Veterinary Surgeons.
7. Godshalk CP, et al: Gastric perforation associated with administration of ibuprofen in a dog. *J Am Vet Med Assoc* 201:1734–1736, 1992.
8. Scherke R, Frey HH: Pharmacokinetics of ibuprofen in the dog. *J Vet Pharmacol Ther* 10:261–265, 1987.
9. Jones RD, Baynes RE, Nimitz CT: Non-steroidal Anti-inflammatory drug toxicosis in dogs and cats: 240 cases (1989–1990). *J Am Vet Med Assoc* 20:No. 3:475–477, 1992.

10. Cataldo PA, Senagore AJ, Kilbride MJ: Ketolorac and patient controlled analgesia in the treatment of postoperative pain. *Surgery Gynecology and Obstetrics* 176:435–438, 1993.
11. Peirce RJ, Fragan RJ, Pemberton DM: Intravenous ketolorac thromethomine versus morphine sulfate in the treatment of immediate postoperative pain. *Pharmacotherapy* 10: 111–115, 1990.
12. Ogen W, et al: *Constant cold therapy for total joint replacements.* Proceeding: Piedmont Orthopaedic Society, May 1990.
13. Thompson SE, Johnson JM: Postoperative analgesia in dogs after intercostal thoracotomy: a comparison of morphine, selective intercostal nerve block, and pleural regional anesthesia with bupivicaine. *Vet Surg* 20:73–77, 1991.

7

Cardiopulmonary Arrest in the Postoperative Patient

S. W. PETERSEN, DVM

Cardiopulmonary arrest may occur in the postoperative patient secondary to a variety of causes, including drug overdose, surgical complication, massive blood loss, preexisting disease, respiratory compromise, or rarely, primary myocardial dysfunction. Ventilatory failure with secondary cerebral and myocardial hypoxia appears to initiate cardiopulmonary arrest more commonly in dogs and cats than does cardiac disease [1]. Therefore, postoperative patients therefore need to be monitored very carefully for return of voluntary respiration and airway patency both before and after endotracheal tube extubation.

Preexisting metabolic disturbances should be corrected before surgery. Intraoperative blood loss should be monitored and corrected as needed during surgery with crytalloid fluids and/or blood products. Long-acting, slowly metabolized, anesthetic agents should be avoided. Critically sick patients that cannot be stabilized adequately before surgery can be induced for anesthesia with mask induction. Intravenous bolus injection of propofol (Diprivan, Stuart Pharmaceuticals, Wilmington, Del.) will allow rapid induction and immediate intubation, with minimal lingering effects because of rapid metabolism [2,3]. A combination of lidocaine and diazepam (Valium, Roche Products, Manabl, Puerto Rico) has been shown to be a cardiosupportive and effective induction agent in critically unstable patients [4].

Resuscitative priorities have not changed in many years and were established originally to focus efforts on basic life-support measures. The *ABCs* of cardiopulmonary resuscitation (CPR) include:

Assess the patient to determine the cause for arrest,
Airway securement,
Breathe for the animal, and
Circulation via closed-chest thoracic compressions.

Diagnosis and Definitive treatment are necessary adjuncts to the *ABC* mantra. It is important to identify the cause of the cardiopulmonary arrest and to treat arrythmias and electrolyte imbalances as they occur.

A thorough but rapid physical examination should be performed to determine the cause of arrest and whether resuscitative efforts should be initiated. Following the examination, or simultaneously, the first priority is to secure a patent airway. Endotracheal intubation is preferred. Most postoperative animals either will still be intubated at the time of arrest or their endotracheal tube will be close at hand. Suction capabilities are helpful in removing blood, mucus, vomitus, or other foreign material that may be obstructing or occluding the upper airway (i.e., oral pharynx and larynx). In rare circumstances, immediate tracheostomy may be needed to provide a patent airway; for example, a patient may suffer acute postoperative laryngeal paralysis secondary to surgery around the cervical trachea.

Once a patent airway has been established, positive-pressure ventilation should be initiated. An oxygen source such as an anesthetic machine with clean hoses will provide 100% oxygen. A self-inflating resuscitation bag that uses room air provides 21% O_2; these bags also may be connected to an O_2 source to provide 100% O_2. Current recommendations are to initiate a breathing pattern and frequency that provide moderate hyperventilation to counteract the metabolic acidosis that develops with cardiopulmonary arrest [1]. Therefore, the familiar pattern of one interposed ventilation per every five thoracic compressions would only provide 12 to 24 breaths/min, which has been shown experimentally to result in development of arterial hypercapnia (i.e., increased arterial carbon dioxide) in a model of cardiopulmonary arrest [4,5]. A ventilatory rate that more closely equals the thoracic rate, such as that achieved with simultaneous compression and ventilation CPR technique, is thus preferred.

Circulation is the next focus of CPR efforts. Cardiac compression is the means by which artificial circulation is achieved during CPR. External cardiac compression (i.e., closed-chest CPR) is the recommended method [1]. Open-chest CPR (i.e., cardiac massage) has fallen out of favor for resuscitation of most cardiac-arrest patients [1]. This technique should be restricted to situations in which intraoperative cardiac arrest occurs and the animal's thorax is already open or in those with penetrating thoracic trauma [1].

A discussion of closed-chest CPR would not be complete without a brief divergence into the physiology behind external cardiac compressions. Two basic premises describe blood flow during CPR: the cardiac-pump theory, and the thoracic-pump theory. The basic thought behind the cardiac-pump theory is that external chest compressions result in direct compressions of the heart, with compression of the ventricles and closing of the atrioventricular valves, which ultimately results in an antegrade flow of blood from the heart. This theory may hold true in cats and small dogs with compliant thoracic walls [1]. The premise behind the thoracic-pump theory is that external chest compressions cause changes in intrathoracic pressure, which forces blood from the thoracic blood vessels into the systemic circulation. In this theory, the heart acts solely as a conduit and not as a pump.

Compression rates have been established based on patient size and correlation with their prearrest resting heart rate. Rates ranging from 60 to 120 compressions/min have been recommended for dogs and cats [1]. Currently, the recommendation for small dogs and cats (body weight, < 15 kg) is 100 to 120 compressions/min [1]. For larger dogs (body weight, > 15 kg), the recommended rate drops to 80 to 100 compressions/min. Irrespective of the patient's weight, attention should be placed on maintaining a compression duration of 50% of the cycle time, which will potentiate blood flow via the thoracic -pump theory (i.e., intrathoracic pressure changes) [1].

The force applied should compress the thoracic cavity by 25% to 30% of its diameter [1]. The most important aspect of body position during CPR is stability of the patient so that adequate thoracic compressions can be delivered. Thus, lateral recumbency has been recommended for animals weighing less than 15 kg and dorsal recumbency for animals greater than 15 kg, but only if this position can be stabilized adequately [1].

Recommendations for artificial respiration include a rate of 20 to 24 breaths/ min with 100% oxygen [1]. Breaths should be interposed between compressions. Simultaneous ventilation/compression techniques, however, have been shown experimentally to result in improved arterial oxygenation [4,5]. The higher ventilatory rates achieved with simultaneous ventilations and compressions may be useful in helping to prevent and/or counteract the development of metabolic acidosis [1,4,5,6].

Adjunctive drug therapy during CPR can be critical to the success of resusscitative efforts. As mentioned previously, 100% oxygen should be administered if available during artificial respirations. Fluid administration during resuscitative efforts should be conservative, unless preexisting hypovolemia has contributed to the arrest [6,7]. The goal of drug therapy is to improve blood flow and, thus, oxygen to the brain and myocardial tissue. Epinephrine is a mixed α- and β-adrenergic agonist that has been commonly used during CPR because of its positive circulatory effects. Studies have investigated the effects of pure α-agonists (e.g., methoxamine, norepinephrine) in CPR; however, these agents have not been proven to be superior to epinephrine [1,6]. The positive hemodynamic effects of epinephrine and other α-agonists [1,6] include:

1. Peripheral vasoconstriction that results in venous return and prevention of arterial collapse,
2. Improved coronary blood flow secondary to increased aortic diastolic pressure, and
3. Increased intracranial blood flow resulting from vasoconstriction of extracranial portions of the carotid artery.

The β-adrenergic effects of epinephrine cause dilation of cerebral microvasculature with resulting improved cerebral tissue perfusion [1,6]. Current recommendations are for high-dose administration of epinephrine (0.2 mg/kg) as the adrenergic agonist of choice [1,6].

The preferred route of drug administration during CPR is intravenous, but studies have not proven that a central venous route is superior to a peripheral venous route [1]. Intraosseous drug administration is a proven alternative and may be especially effective in smaller animals, neonates, and pocket pets [8,9,10]. Endotracheal administration with transalveolar absorption is another alternative for epinephrine, atropine, and lidocaine [6]. This route may be indicated with patients that do not have a secure intravenous line.

Assessment of cardiac function and recognition of arrythmias are important aspects of successful resuscitative efforts. Detection of cardiac arrythmias is best accomplished with electrocardiogram (ECG) monitoring and physical examination (peripheral pulse palpation). The most commonly identified arrythmias during cardiopulmonary arrest in dogs and cats, in order of frequency detected, include electromechanical dissociation, ventricular asystole, ventricular fibrillation, and sinus bradycardia.

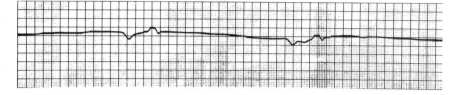

Fig. 7–1. Electrocardiographic tracing of electromechanical dissociation. (With permission from Edwards NJ: Electromechanical dissociation. *In Bolton's handbook of canine and feline electrocardiography,* edn 2. Philadelphia, 1977, WB Saunders.)

Electromechanical dissociation is a condition in which normal cardiac electrical patterns, P waves, and/or QRS complexes are visible on the ECG but peripheral arterial pulses are absent [6,7] (Fig. 7–1). Thus, as the name implies, the heart is functioning electrically but not mechanically, and no arterial pulses are generated. Treatment recommendations for EMD include high-dose epinephrine (0.2 mg/kg intravenously) or high doses of dexamethasone sodium phosphate (4.0 mg/kg intravenously) [6,7]. Resuscitative efforts should be continued as outlined previously. Prognosis for resuscitation from electromechanical dissociation is generally poor for animals with underlying cardiac or metabolic disease. If this condition results from a physical disorder such as postoperative pneumothorax or cardiac tamponade, the prognosis for recovery is much better with correction of the initiating condition.

Ventricular asystole, or "flat line," is probably the most easily recognized arrythmia (Fig. 7–2). An ECG tracing will reveal a total absence of QRS-T complexes. Recommendations for treatment include high-dose epinephrine (0.2 mg/kg intravenously) combined with continued CPR efforts [6,7]. Atropine (0.04 mg/kg intravenously) may be especially helpful if the ventricular asystole is secondary to excessive vagal stimulation [6,7].

Ventricular fibrillation, or "V-fib," has been described as the most common cause of acute death in dogs and cats suffering from cardiac arrest[7] (Fig. 7–3). This

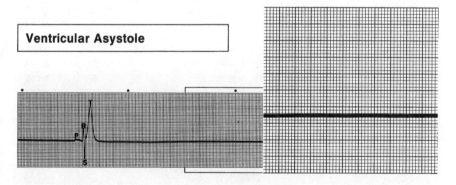

Fig. 7–2. Ventricular asystole. It is important that all of the electrocardiographic leads are properly applied and good patient contact made to avoid misdiagnosis of this problem. (From Tilley, L.P.: Essentials of Canine and Feline Electrocardiography. St. Louis, C.V. Mosby Co. 1979.)

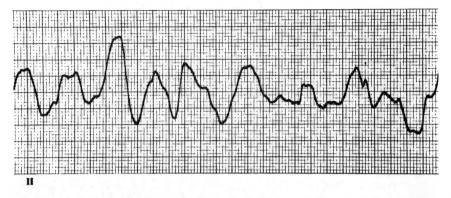

Fig. 7–3.   Ventricular fibrillation. (With permission from Edwards NJ: Electromechanical dissociation. *In Bolton's handbook of canine and feline electrocardiography,* edn 2. Philadelphia, 1977, WB Saunders.)

condition is recognized on ECG by the presence of coarse or fine, unorganized fibrillation waves and the absence of identifiable QRS-T complexes. The heart is contracting asynchronously, and cardiac output drops to nil. The treatment of choice for ventricular fibrillation is immediate defibrillating electrical shock [7]; chemical defibrillation is of questionable efficacy [7]. Administration of lidocaine appears to be contraindicated, because it may increase the defibrillation threshold and thus decrease the success of electrical defibrillation [7].

Sinus bradycardia is the fourth most commonly recognized arrythmia in cardiac-arrest patients [7] (Fig. 7–4). Postoperative hypothermia and residual anesthetic agents are recognized as causes of this condition. Other cardiac drugs and increased vagal tone also can produce sinus bradycardia. Heart rates under 60 bpm for dogs and 140 bpm for cats are consistent with sinus bradycardia [7]. Atropine (0.04 mg/kg intravenously) is the drug of choice when bradycardia results from excessive vagal tone. Sympathomimetic drugs such as epinephrine (0.2 mg/kg intravenously) are recommended for treating bradycardia associated with hypothermia, drugs, anesthetic agents, or in animals undergoing cardiac arrest [7]. A constant-rate infusion of dopamine (5–20 μg/kg/min intravenously) is also effective in correcting sinus bradycardia and improving cardiac output in the postoperative patient.

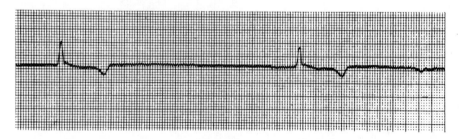

Fig. 7–4.   Severe bradycardia in a patient suffering from hypothermia. (With permission from Edwards NJ: Electromechanical dissociation. *In Bolton's handbook of canine and feline electrocardiography,* edn 2. Philadelphia, 1977, WB Saunders.)

As a concluding thought, even though CPR has been used in human and veterinary medicine for many years to treat cardiopulmonary arrest, the overall success rate is disappointing. As one author described, it is "a desperate effort that will help only a limited number of patients" [1]. This does not imply that CPR efforts should not be attempted. Rather, it reinforces the goal to prevent cardiopulmonary arrest from occuring initially.

REFERENCES

1. Nieman JT: Cardiopulmonary resuscitation—current concepts. *N Engl J Med* 327: 1075–1080, 1992.
2. Robertson SA, Johnston S, Beemsterboer J: Cardiopulmonary, anesthetic, and postanesthetic effects of intravenous infusions of propofol in greyhounds and non-greyhounds. *Am J Vet Res* 53(G):1027–1032, 1992.
3. Ilkin JE, et al: Cardiovascular and respiratory effects of propofol administration in hypovolemic dogs. *Am J Vet Res* 53:2323–2327, 1992.
4. Henik RA: Basic life support and external cardiac compression in dogs and cats. *J Am Vet Med* 200:1925–1931 1992.
5. Henrik RA: Effects of body position and ventilation/compression ratios during cardiopulmonary resuscitation in cats. *Am J Vet Res* 48:1603–1606, 1987.
6. Vanpelt DR, Wingfield WE: Controversial issues in drug treatment during cardiopulmonary resuscitation. *J Am Vet Med Assoc* 200:1938–1944, 1992.
7. Rush JE, Wingfield WE: Recognition and frequency of disrythmmias during cardiopulmonary arrest. *J Am Vet Med Assoc* 200:1932–1937, 1992.
8. Brickman KR, Rega P, Guinness M. A comparative study of intraosseous versus peripheral intravenous infusion of diazepam and phenobarbital in dogs. *Ann Emerg Med* 16: 1141–1144, 1987.
9. Hodge D, Delgado C, Fleisher C. Intraosseous infusion flow rates in hypovolemic "pediatric" dogs. *Ann Emerg Med* 16(3):101, 1987.
10. Okrasinski EB, Krahwinkel DJ. Treatment of dogs in hemorrhagic shock by intraosseous infusion of hypertonic saline and dextran. *J Vet Surg* 21(1):20–24, 1992.
11. Bjorling DE, Rawlings CA. Induction of anesthesia with thiopental-lidocaine combination in dogs with cardiopulmonary disease. *J Am Aml Hosp Assoc* vol 20 p 445–448, 1984.

8

Postanesthetic Recovery Care

LISA LEE, BS, CVT

Induction of and recovery from anesthesia are periods of extreme risk, as the respective depression and arousal of the central nervous system (CNS) impacts critical physiologic functions. While induction typically initiates close monitoring of these functions, there is a tendency to become less vigilant as the animal recovers. In many practices, the purchase and supply of monitoring equipment is more heavily shifted toward the operating room rather than the recovery area. In addition, parameters such as heart rate, blood pressure, and respiration that are assessed and documented every 5 minutes beginning with induction are often discontinued as the animal is disconnected from anesthetic administration. The scenario of witnessing or performing efficient diagnosis, stabilization, and life-saving surgical technique on an animal only to see it lost to an easily prevented complication such as airway obstruction is painfully familiar to many experienced veterinary professionals. Most postoperative problems that are described as complications of general anesthesia usually result from preexisting disease and magnitude of the surgical procedure. An 8% to 10% complication rate in 112,000 anesthetic procedures has been reported in humans; however, the incidence of life-threatening complications was less than 1% [1].

METABOLISM AND EXCRETION OF INHALANT ANESTHETICS

Excretion of inhalant anesthetics is achieved by exhalation. As the anesthetic flow is reduced, the partial pressure of the gas becomes higher in the venous blood than the alveoli, and diffusion from pulmonary capillaries to the lungs for exhalation occurs. Anesthetic diffusion from tissues then follows as the arterial levels drop. All inhalant anesthetics are thus exhaled, but the rate and extent of this process is determined by the individual agent's solubility.

Solubility also can be expressed in terms of the ratio of anesthetic to other solvents such as fat (Table 8–1). In this case, high coefficients delay recovery because of the expanse of adipose (10% to 30% of body mass) [2] and its high proclivity for absorbing anesthetic versus its poor capabilities of metabolism and anesthetic removal via diffusion. Fat receives only approximately 5% of cardiac output [2]. In

Table 8–1
Gas Coefficients for Common Anesthetic Agents

	Partition Coefficient	
Anesthetic	Blood/Gas*	Fat/Blood
Methoxyflurane	13.0	61.0
Halothane	2.36	65.0
Enflurane	1.91	37.0
Isoflurane	1.41	48.1
Nitrous Oxide	0.49	2.3

* A blood/gas coefficient of 2.0 would express a ratio of one volume of anesthetic in the alveoli to two voumes of gas in the blood at equilibrium.
From *Handbook of veterinary anesthesia:* St. Louis, 1989, pp. 91–92 Mosby–Year Book.

absorbing anesthetic, fat increases the amount of hepatic biotransformation and renal excretion necessary for elimination of the drug. The high fat solubility of methoxyflurane, for example, may result in the presence of this compound in the blood as late as 24 hours after clinical recovery [3]. Approximately 50% of the uptake of this agent may require metabolism, compared with 10% to 20% of halothane, 2.5% of enflurane, and 0.25% of isoflurane [2]. An understanding of elimination and metabolic requisites is important, however, considering that the fraction of anesthetic exhaled by the animal in recovery represents potential human exposure.

The liver transforms lipid-soluble anesthetics to water-soluble agents. This is important in that fat-soluble agents more readily cross cell membranes but are more slowly excreted. Once biotransformed, the water-soluble agent is conjugated to an organic acid for excretion. The higher the rate of liver metabolism of a drug, the more important hepatic blood flow becomes. Drugs metabolized more slowly by the liver are more affected by enzyme activity. Diazepam and acepromazine are common examples of the latter, whereas morphine and meperidine would be impacted by hepatic blood supply [4]. In the case of methoxyflurane, the fraction of gas not exhaled results in toxic by-products that may cause kidney damage. A fraction of halothane also is metabolized by the liver; whether oxidation or reduction occurs regarding its metabolism determines the toxicity of the by-products.

BARBITURATE RECOVERY

Elimination of barbiturates is affected by such factors as blood and tissue pH, redistribution to nonervous tissue, type of agent used, and rate of liver detoxification and renal excretion. Because these agents cannot be reversed overdose is a major cause of deaths from anesthesia in small animals [5], a basic understanding of their metabolim is paramount. Barbiturates are administered as sodium salts that enter the brain and other lipid-cell membranes in an nonionized form. If the body undergoes any lowering of pH, more of the drug's nonionized form is present in the bloodstream to cross membranes such as those of the CNS. This has the effect of greater CNS depression, which results in greater respiratory depression. Hypercarbia resulting from the respiratory depression causes respiratory acidosis and reduced blood pH if allowed to go unchecked. The more acidic environment of the blood then increases the effect of the drug. Also, the CNS becomes more depressed, and a negative cycle of respiratory depression is possible unless ventilatory support is provided. Recovery staff should be alerted to prolonged or profound depression when these agents have been used, particularly if intraoperative conditions suggest acidemia or hypoproteinemia because of severe hemorrhage or plasma loss. Ventilatory support and acid–base determinations may be required to prevent further CNS depression.

Barbiturate metabolism actually may be influenced more by anesthetic redistribution than by biotransformation and excretion. Recovery is based on a drop in plasma concentration below the level of CNS depression and occurs because of redistribution to muscle and then to fat. This is followed by passive diffusion of the barbiturate from higher levels in the brain to the reduced levels in the blood. As opposed to the case of inhalant anesthetics, the higher lipid solubility in barbiturates creates a more rapid redistribution and immediate recovery, while agents of decreased fat solubility primarily require liver metabolism and kidney excretion. Thiobarbiturates such as thiamylal and thiopental are more fat redistributed and thus very short acting, while oxybarbiturates such as pentobarbital are longer acting because of reduced fat redistribution and metabolic requisite.

Body fat composition also may influence metabolism, particularly if repeat doses of thiobarbiturates are administered [5]. In this case, emaciated animals or lean breeds experience a prolonged recovery because of an inadequate supply of redistributive reservoir. In contrast, obese animals may regain reflexes sooner but exhibit prolonged elimination of anesthetic because of adipose-tissue residue. Hypovolemic animals will have difficulty redistributing barbiturates, because their cardiac output is being diverted to the vital organs. This and other reduction in the blood supply to muscle and fat may result in overdose or severe CNS depression during recovery. In view of the availability of so many other anesthetic agents available, use of barbiturates in hypotensive or very lean animals is contraindicated when choosing an anesthetic regimen.

INJECTABLE PREANESTHETIC AND INDUCTION AGENTS

Liver enzyme biotransformation must occur to terminate the barbiturate effect; this enzyme function is reduced when hypothermia is present. In contrast, repeat dosing with barbiturates actually may increase enzyme levels and thus hasten recovery [4,6]. The rapid rate of hepatic metabolism renders methohexital sodium; an ultrashort-acting agent of 25- to 30-minute duration, even though it is poorly redistributed [5]. In healthy animals, the process of removing the active form of barbiturates and excreting their metabolites occurs in approximately 6 to 8 hours [5]. Animals with compromised hepatic and/or renal function are poor candidates for these agents and, at best, will experience a prolonged recovery.

DISSOCIATIVE RECOVERY

Ketamine hydrochloride often is used as a sole anesthetic agent for minor procedures in cats and in combination with other premedicating or induction agents in a number of animal species. Ketamine is lipid soluble and distributes to all body tissues; there usually is a rapid drop in plasma levels soon after injection because of this distribution, followed by a slower drop over a 4- to 8-hour period [7]. The duration of effect following intravenous administration is approximately 3 to 10 minutes, compared with 20 to 30 minutes when given intamuscularly in the dog and 30 to 60 minutes in the cat [4]. Complete recovery from ketamine occurs in approximately 1 to 3 hours when given intravenously and 4 to 6 hours when given intramuscularly [5]. It should be noted that extreme variance in recovery occurs when ketamine is administered intramuscularly in cats, and some animals may take 24 hours or longer to recover [5]. In dogs, ketamine undergoes biotransformation by the liver with the water-soluble metabolites excreted in the urine. In cats, however, 87% of the drug is excreted in the active, unmetabolized form [8]. Particular attention thus should be paid to urine output, renal function, and signs of urinary obstruction in feline ketamine recovery.

ENVIRONMENTAL CONCERNS

The principles of excretion and metabolism of inhalation anesthetics render adequate ventilation of the recovery area important to minimize exposure of medical personnel to waste-gas pollution. In addition to toxic metabolite effects, general exposure to anesthetics has been correlated with mutagenicity, carcinogenicity [9–11], and dermatitis in the case of halothane [11]. Nitrous oxide has been implicated specifically as being associated with polyneuropathy and reduced cell-mediated immune response [12].

To maintain air quality below the maximum limits set by the National Institute for Occupational Safety and Health (NIOSH), halogenated hydrocarbons such as halothane, isoflurane, and methoxyflurane must be kept below 2.0 ppm; below 0.5 ppm if used with N_2O; and below 25.0 ppm if N_2O alone is used [4,5,9–11]. At least 10 total air exchanges per hour are required by general ventilation to achieve these standards [5]; however, scavenging systems are a much more effective means of controlling waste gas and have been found to dramatically reduce waste-gas concentrations during anesthesia. Scavenging systems essentially direct collected gases from the work area or exhalation components of the anesthetic machine through a closed transport to an area avoiding exposure of medical personnel. Unfortunately, the recovery area represents a high potential for contamination, because the extubated animal expires into an open system (i.e., room air) that cannot be scavenged directly. In one controlled study of recovery-room gas concentrations following anesthesia of 36 dogs, anesthetic concentrations were found to exceed those recommended by the NIOSH [10]. Minimization of direct patient-contact time and frequency of air exchanges were cited as methods to reduce personnel risk [10].

In addition to waste-gas recovery, sanitation is critical, as the volume and transience of the recovery area represent a high potential for wound contamination or systemic infection. General anesthesia itself may compound this potential because of immune-mediated depression by agents such as thiobarbiturates and halothane [13].

PREDISPOSING FACTORS IN CARDIOPULMONARY ARREST

Primary predisposing factors to cardiopulmonary arrest are trauma in cats and respiratory pathology in dogs [14]. Any condition that produces cellular hypoxia may cause cardiac dysfunctions. Examples of these encountered postanesthetically are airway obstructions, such as a kink or mucus plug in the endotracheal tube; vasoconstriction secondary to hypotension or hypothermia; and a decreased percentage of inspired oxygen as the animal is disconnected from O_2 and gas. Other conditions predisposing an animal to cardiopulmonary arrest are acidemia, electrolyte imbalances, and cerebral or thoracic contusions.

The importance of preventing cardiopulmonary arrest highlights the need for communication by the intraoperative team if the animal has sustained predisposing pathology during the surgical procedure. In addition, the recovery team must be prepared for early detection of the signs of impending arrest (Table 8–2). If signs are detected, electrocardiography should be used to more accurately determine cardiac function. A Doppler or other means of determining accurate blood pressure also should be used.

In the absence of such capability, general parameters may prove useful. An arterial pulse is palpbable at greater than 70 mm Hg [15]. Peripheral pulse is undetectable below a systolic blood pressure of 60 mm Hg. Below a systolic blood pressure of 50 mm Hg, heart sounds are undeterminable [14].

HYPOXIA

There are several postanesthetic causes of hypoxia [16]. These are:

1. A decrease in inspired O_2 fraction,
2. An increased and uncompensated need for supplemental O_2,
3. Alveolar hypoventilation,
4. Diffusion dysfunction,
5. Ventilation–perfusion (V/Q) mismatching, and
6. Anatomic shunt.

Table 8–2
Warning Signs and Predisposing Factors to Cardiopulmonary Arrest
during Recovery

Warning Signs in Recovery	Predisposing Factors
Weak pulse	Anesthetic overdose
Irregular pulse	Inadequate ventilation
Respiratory rate changes	Preexisting disease
Respiratory volume changes	
Change in mucous membrane color	
Relapse of consciousness level	
Drop in body temperature	
Long periods of hypotension	
Anaphylactoid reaction to anesthetic agent	
Progressive bradycardia	

Levels of FIo_2 refer to the fractional percentage of O_2 inhaled. Room air has been analyzed as having 20.93% O_2 [17] and thus has an FIo_2 level of approximately 0.21 as opposed to anesthetic O_2, which is supplied at 100% and thus has an FIo_2 rating of 1.0. This represents a stark contrast to the animal in terms of adapting to the transfer from supplemental anesthetic flows to that of inspired room air.

While most patients are able to compensate for this reduction, those with systemic disease and cardiac or pulmonary dysfunction may require maintenance of artificially high FIo_2 levels if hypoxia is to be avoided. In some cases, hypoxia is created by an intrinsically increased demand for O_2 that is not recognized or compensated for in recovery. Shivering, for example, represents a marked increase in muscle activity and demand for O_2; if previously depressed and taxed cardiopulmonary systems cannot keep up with these demands, hypoxia may result. Animals with a burn injury also may represent a hypermetabolic recovery state, the degree of which is proportional to the size and severity of the trauma [18]. Postanesthetic O_2 also should be offered to such cases in that pulmonary shunting is more likely increased as well in this type of trauma [18].

Alveolar hypoventilation refers to a decrease of fresh inspired air per breathing interval, and it is associated with concurrently elevated $Paco_2$ levels. This is the most common cause of iatrogenic hypoxia because of probability and, in some cases, insidious onset. General anesthetics, narcotics, barbiturates, and CNS depression such as hypothermia depress the respiratory control center and represent the probable aspect of postanesthetic hypoventilation. Airway obstruction and conditions precluding effective ventilation are more acute causes of recovery hypoventilation.

In diffusion dysfunction, there is an increase in the barrier through which O_2 must pass to reach hemoglobin. If normal barriers such as the alveolar epithelium, capillary membrane, and endothelium [16] are thickened or inflamed, diffusion of O_2 may be effectively reduced. Pulmonary parenchymal disease such as pneumonia and pulmonary edema represent examples of this hypoxia etiology. The V/Q ratio represents that of alveolar ventilation to pulmonary blood flow; when this ratio differs from that of established normal parameters, V/Q mismatch occurs. Therefore, it is important to recognize that both alveolar ventilation and transfer of gases at the pulmonary perfusion level are important in maintaining normal Pao_2/$Paco_2$ levels during recovery.

Determining the primary cause of the hypoxia is important in assessing the value of treatment with O_2. For example, hypoxia associated with alveolar hypoventilation diffusion impairment and, in some cases, V/Q mismatching may be alleviated with 100% O_2 [16]. Anatomic shunting such as that occurring in congenital heart disease does not respond to increased FIo_2 levels, because blood bypassed the supplemental O_2 increase in the alveoli. If blood-gas measures are available, Pao_2 levels below 75 mm Hg indicate a need for increased O_2 [19], and levels below 60 mm Hg indicate a need for aggressive ventilatory therapy [4]. In the absence of blood-gas analysis, clinical signs such as dyspnea, retraction of the oral commissure, tachycardia, arrythmias, gastrointestinal upset, and ataxia may be used as indicators of the need for O_2 therapy.

PULSE OXIMETRY

Pulse oximetry is a noninvasive technique whereby light is passed through tissue, detecting the uptake of oxyhemoglobin and thus measuring Sao_2 levels. A red and infrared light-emitting lead is passed over a vascular bed, and O_2 saturation is measured by the intensity of the light transmitted to a photodetector. The premise is that oxyhemoglobin and deoxyhemoglobin have fixed patterns of absorption for this spectrum of light. Because of vascularity and positional convenience, the tongue and nasal septum represent the best position for the monitor lead. Pulse oximetry is sensitive to reduced pulse volume caused by severe blood loss or vasoconstriction. Excessive environmental lighting, bilirubinemia, severe anemia, or hemodilution also may cause inaccurate measures.

Because one of the most preventative complications in recovery is hypoxia, monitoring patient oxygenation through pulse oximetry is essential. The percentage of hemoglobin saturated with O_2 is normally 95% to 98% [20], with higher levels expected in an animal inspiring enriched O_2. A decrease below 90% Sao_2 [20] is associated with a marked decrease in O_2 delivery to tissues despite a small decrease in O_2 tension resulting from a nonlinear shape of the Sao_2/Po_2 curve. Saturation is of high clinical significance, because 95% of O_2 delivery to tissues is by oxyhemoglobin [20]. Decreased delivery of O_2 to vital organs may precede collapse and, to other tissues, may result in lactic acidosis and metabolic abnormalities.

Correlation of end-tidal CO_2 levels ($ETco_2$) and SaO_2 levels can be helpful in diagnosing and correcting inadequate perfusion. Normal values should indicate $ETco_2$ levels between 35 and 45 mm Hg and Sao_2 levels above 90%. Elevated $ETco_2$ levels associated with decreased Sao_2 levels often indicate hypoventilation and may be corrected with assisted ventilation. Inadequate response to this corrective effort often indicates V/Q mismatch; this is the most common cause of hypoxia in critical patients [20]. Strictured airways, vascular anomaly, and inadequate alveolar filling are common causes, and differential diagnosis with appropriate corrective efforts should be made.

OXYGEN ADMINISTRATION

Because O_2 is required for cell oxidation and energy production, anoxia represents tissue death and organ dysfunction in the body. The goal of O_2 therapy is to prevent further tissue damage and reverse whatever negative processes that can be. Fortunately, pathology such as respiratory depression as a cause of hypoxia during recovery may be self-limiting when preanesthetic equilibrium is reestablished. In this case, supplemental O_2 is offered as a supportive measure to decrease workload on the cardiopulmonary system and sustain systemic homeostatic efforts. If the need for increased O_2 is mild, FIo_2 levels of 0.3 to 0.4 typically are adequate to prevent hypoxia; more severe cases may require FIo_2 levels of 0.5 or more [16]. Animals maintained at FIo_2 levels over 0.5 for more than 24 hours may develop pulmonary pathology [16]. Prolonged exposure to 100% O_2 causes both acute and chronic changes in pulmonary anatomy and physiology. Acutely, necrosis of the pulmonary endothelium and alveolar lining may occur. In the chronic stage, fibrous thickening and exudative changes in pulmonary tissue may occur and result in diffusion deficits [5,16].

If the animal is still intubated in the recovery area, O_2 may be supplemented via the endotracheal tube; this may be achieved by several direct methods. The animal can be maintained on O_2 via anesthetic equipment at 30 mL/kg of body weight on a rebreathing system or 200 mL/kg on a nonrebreathing system. This technique is not recommended if soluble anesthetics have been used because of anesthetic residuals in the rubber tubing. Many manual ventilators have ports for an augmentative O_2 line. This O_2 mixes with room air in the reservoir bag and increases the FIo_2 level. The tube also may be insufflated with O_2 at 2 to 3 L/min [19]; this method is ideal in its reduction of both mechanical and physiologic dead space. After extubation, methods of O_2 administration include masks, nasal catheters, transtracheal catheterization, and O_2 cages. Masks of different sizes are available for small animals. Eye ointment should be placed in the animal's eyes to prevent dessication. Oxygen is delivered at 8 to 12 L/min to maintain an FIo_2 of 1.0 [16]. Although this route is easy and effective, it has the disadvantages of requiring restraint and high flow rates, and it represents a high degree of mechanical dead space in terms of supply economy. Nasal catheters offer less restraint requisite but may cause gastric dilatation and volvulus if placed too far distal in the pharynx. In this method, local anesthetic drops are placed in the nare, and a soft, red-rubber catheter is passed via the nose into the proximal pharynx. The catheter should be fenestrated and an Elizabethan collar used to prevent extraction by the animal. The flow of O_2 is delivered at 6 to 8 L/min [16].

Acceptance of supplementation is higher with transtracheal catheterization and O_2 cages, and these methods are indicated for long-term therapy. In transtracheal catheterization, percutaneous entry into the trachea is made through the cricoid ligament. This landmark is found by locating the trangular depression just superior to the cricoid cartilage when the animal's neck is extended. A 14- to 16-G intravenous catheter that has been fenestrated with distal grooves is inserted, and the stylet is removed. Tape is looped around the catheter and the animal's neck, and flow rates are maintained at 3 to 6 L/min depending on the animal's size [21]. The primary disadvantage of this method is the tissue invasion and potential for infection if sterile technique is not applied. Also, the O_2 cage offers good control but is expensive in terms of O_2 flow as well as initial purchase. The cage should be flushed for 1 to 5 minutes at 30 to 40 L/min and then may be maintained at 5 L/min at a FIo_2 level of 1.0 [16].

The recovery team should be aware that O_2 therapy may bypass or inhibit function of the upper airway in filtering, warming, and moistening inspired gases. Aside from O_2 toxicity, sequelae that may occur from supplementation include thickened secretions, decreased mucociliary function, retention of secretions, inflammation, shunting and hyperthermia. Flowmeters and O_2 cages should be used during recovery to minimize the negative effects on respiratory functional anatomy.

EXPIRED GAS VALUES AND APPLICATION

End-tidal CO_2 is the concentration of CO_2 in a sample of airway gas at the end of respiration. This value may be taken noninvasively by sampling at the mouth or nares. $ETco_2$ is a useful parameter in that it directly reflects alveolar and arterial CO_2 ($Paco_2$) levels as long as tachypnea (>60 breaths/min) and no serious pulmonary disease such as obstruction or shunting are present [20].

Normally, the medullary respiratory centers keep $Paco_2$ levels at approximately 40 mm Hg and within a range of 35 to 45 mm Hg [22]. Normal $ETco_2$ levels thus can be expected to be within these limits. Levels greater than 45 mm Hg suggest hypoventilation with or without V/Q mismatch. At levels of 50 mm Hg or more, respiratory acidosis ensues because of the excessive formation of carbonic acid and its subsequent dissociation and hydrogen ion formation. Levels of 60 mm Hg or more represent a hypercarbia capable of producing life-threatening acidemia [22]. If the animal is breathing room air, associated P_{O_2} levels would be anticipated to cause hypoxemia, because an increase in Pa_{CO_2} would cause an approximately equivalent and paradoxic decrease in Pa_{O_2} levels. Aggressive ventilatory therapy thus is indicated at this level. ET_{CO_2} levels less than 35 reflect hyperventilation; levels below 20 mm Hg are associated with life-threatening respiratory alkalosis as cerebral blood flow and oxygenation may be impaired [22].

End-tidal volume monitors are equipped with alarms that sound when levels of expired gases or respiration rates exceed normal limitations. When allowed to default to automatic settings, the average boundaries on such monitors would be an apnea no greater than 40 seconds and ET_{CO_2} greater than 45 mm Hg for the average of the first eight breaths taken [23]. The latter value is baseline related, but limitations may be set manually to fixed values such as to ET_{CO_2} of 35 to 45 mm Hg.

RESPIRATORY SUPPORT

The concept of maximizing the animal's own ventilatory efforts in recovery is seemingly obvious, but it is commonly overlooked. Efforts to do so may prevent life-threatening conditions that commonly occur in recovery. For example, suctioning chest drains at adequate intervals not only will offer relief in terms of the animal's own respiratory efforts but maintenance that is critical in the prevention of iatrogenic pneumothorax. Thoracic bandages should be checked periodically to ensure that diaphragmatic restriction is not occurring. The patient should be rotated every 15 minutes to prevent hypostatic congestion unless it is surgically contraindicated, because hypostatic congestion of a lung field may occur in 30 to 45 minutes [5]. Prolonged recumbency also may impair respiration or cause tissue hypoxia, particularly in the obese patient.

AIRWAY OBSTRUCTION

The airway should be cleared, and suctioned if necessary, for mucous secretions or debris. Airway obstruction is likely during the recovery period, because pharyngeal reflex may not yet be reestablished. In addition, surgical or mechanical obstructions such as postoperative pharyngeal swelling and occluded endotracheal tubes may result in complications. Brachycephalics are at high risk for obstruction because of stenotic nares [24], soft-palate occlusion, and aerophagic-induced vomiting [19]. In such breeds, the endotracheal tube should be maintained as long as possible. Fentanyl is a nonemetic narcotic that may aid in this retention. An intravenous dose of 0.005 mg/kg is typically adequate and may be reversed with nalaxone when narcotization is no longer warranted. When extubated, the animal's color and respiratory sounds should be monitored closely. Reintubation or mechanical support of the soft palate may be necessary if signs of restricted airflow are evident.

General anesthetic stimulation of the vomition center of the brain may result in postanesthetic emesis and subsequent tracheal occlusion. The chemoreceptor trigger zone in the brain responds to chemicals such as anesthetics agents and anticholinergics, inflammation, osmolality changes, and pyloric distention. There is some evidence that peritoneal and mesenteric vasculature also stimulate emesis [25]. In each case, emesis occurs via facilitation by the vomiting center of the brain [25]. If gastric contents of a low pH are aspirated, pneumonitis is a likely sequela and may require steroidal, antibiotic, and/or respiratory therapy. Animals vomiting in recovery should be attended to by manual clearing of the pharynx, postural drainage, and suctioning. Clearly, prevention is essential regarding this complication. Deflating the endotracheal-tube cuff as the lungs are simultaneously inflated may assist in moving debris lodged at the cuff cranially [19]. In addition, extubating the animal at the end of inspiration leaves expiration as the only respiratory choice, thus reducing the likelihood of aspiration.

HYPOTENSION

The normal mean arterial blood pressure is 90 to 100 mm Hg in the dog and the cat, with a normal systolic range of 135 to 160 mm Hg and a diastolic range of 65 to 80 mm Hg [4]. Deep, general-inhalant anesthesia may reduce the mean arterial pressure by as much as 30 mm Hg [4]. Hypotension occurs during anesthesia, because all anesthetics are negatively inotropic to some degree. Anesthetics may impair autoregulatory mechanisms of blood flow to specific organs as well. Below an arterial pressure of 70 mm Hg, autoregulation is inactive [5], and renal necrosis may occur if this pressure is sustained for over 12 to 24 hours [15]. At pressures below 45 to 50 mm Hg, signs of CNS depression begin to occur; if allowed to persist at levels of 35 mm Hg for over 2 hours, irreversible brain damage will occur [15].

The recovery team should be alert for signs of perfusion inadequacy, such as a weak peripheral pulse, prolonged capillary refill time, tachycardia, pale mucous membranes, and altered levels of consciousness. In addition, an awareness of the conditions and agents that may contribute to hypotension is important in the anticipation and prevention of resultant tissue hypoxia (Table 8–3).

CARDIAC ARRYTHMIAS

Hypoxia, hypotension, acidemia, hypothermia, surgical manipulation, certain induction agents such as thiobarbiturates and xylazine, or anticholinergics may predispose an animal to arrhythmias. Severe trauma cases such as patients hit by a car should be considered as predisposed to arrhythmias because of tramatic myocarditis [26].

Most ventricular arrhythmias such as premature ventricular contractions can be corrected by improving ventilatory status or offering supplemental O_2. The staff should be aware of the animal's anesthetic regimen regarding its potential for arrhythmia.

If arrhythmias were treated intraoperatively with lidocaine or procainamide, recovery care should include monitoring tissue perfusion, electrocardiographic rhythm, effective pulse, and antiarrhythmic drip rate. Tremors or convulsions may occur with lidocaine toxicity, and the drip rate should be reduced or another agent used if these signs are noted. It should be noted that lidocaine potentiates anesthetic effect

Table 8–3
Predisposing Factors in Hypotension

Agents
  Phenothiazines
  Oxymorphone, morphine, meperidine
  Deep-inhalation anesthesia
  Potassium penicillin-G or sodium penicillin-G
  Gentamicin or cephalothin given quickly intravenously
  Barbiturates
  Blood/plasma reaction
Conditions
  Inadequate electrolyte or fluid maintenance during anesthesia
  Preexisting cardiac disease
  Fluid loss without replacement (e.g., high tissue exposure)
  Intrabdominal pressure occluding vena caval return (e.g., GDV)
  High pressure in anesthetic system (e.g., "pop off" valve closed down)
  Tension pneumothorax
  Prolonged inspiratory time during assisted or controlled ventilation (blocking venous
    return)
  Ruptured diaphragmatic hernia repair
  Contrast media leak in radiographic studies

GDV = Gastric Dilatation-Volvulus

and at high doses may cause CNS depression. Animals therefore should be checked continuously for spontaneous recovery signs and possible CNS depression.

NEUROLOGICAL RECOVERY EVENTS

The neurologic changes evident during recovery are consistent with a reversal of the progressive stages leading to surgical anesthesia. Of particular importance is the return of baseline autonomic functions such as cardiovascular tone, respiration, and thermoregulation. As the animal reaches a lighter surgical plane because of the cessation of inhalant delivery, heart rate increases to 90 to 120 bpm (higher in cats) and blood pressure increaeses. Respiration increases to 12 to 20 breaths/min but may fluctuate according to stimulus and blood-gas levels. Muscle tone reappears, as does palpebral reflex and muscle tone. The eyeball rotates medially, then becomes central. As CNS depression lifts, the thermoregulatory center resumes its function, and the animal begins to shiver. This is a normal physiologic response to the hypothermia caused by anesthesia. This increased muscle activity consumes arterial oxygen supply, however, and steps should be taken to warm the animal.

As reflexes return, licking and spastic tongue movements occur. This is the stage of recovery where an animal will attempt to chew and swallow its endotracheal tube. For this reason, an animal should be extubated immediately after the swallowing reflex returns, unless it has not had food withheld overnight or is a brachycephalic breed. Soon after the reflex returns, the animal attempts to right itself. This begins with sternal recumbency and progresses to weight bearing first on the thoracic and then the pelvic limbs. Any delay in normal recovery signs should be noted and weighed against predisposing factors such as hypothermia, obesity, and the use of drugs that prolong recovery.

EMERGENCE DELERIUM

As an animal backs through the stages of anesthesia, it may temporarily undergo a period of hypersensitivity parallel to that of the excitatory stage of induction. Animals are often delerious and may vocalize, paddle uncontrollably, attempt to venture, and hallucinate. The dysphoria involved in this stage of "emergence delerium" may result in musculoskeletal trauma, dehiscence, surgical affectation, and compromised safety of the medical personnel. The duration and degree of reactivity varies according to the animal and the agents used. For example, use of cyclohexamines as induction agents may exacerbate this stage because of CNS dissociation and stimulation. Tranquilizers are effective in reducing the hyperactivity both during induction and recovery; for the systemically depressed animal, sedation may not be an option. In general, patience and attendance often are enough for both the animal and the recovery staff to endure this difficult period. Stimulus minimization, peripheral padding, and prevention of trauma are key components in the safety of the animal as well as the staff. A reasonably quiet recovery environment should be maintained, particularly if the animal is experiencing narcotic auditory sensitization.

THERMOREGULATORY PATHOLOGY

In addition to trauma management, a positive recovery must include efforts toward postanesthetic euthermia. The CNS typically resumes this function as the depression of this system subsides. Unfortunately, in small animals, this often occurs long after a significant change in core temperature has taken place. Wide surgical preparation, large areas of tissue and volume exposure, cold fluids and surgical tables, and nonrebreathed O_2/gas systems may contribute to hypothermia resulting from thermoregulatory depression. Thus, it is not surprising that body temperature as low as 35° C (i.e., 95° F) after 60 to 90 minutes of anesthesia are possible [5]. Animals that are particularly sensitive to hypothermia are geriatrics, neonates, lean breeds, and those with organ failure, large wounds, or infections. In addition to these intraoperative factors, elements of recovery such as the use of narcotics and tranquilizers, reduced muscle activity in the recumbent animal, caloric deficits in the young or fasted animal, and heat loss from large or granulating wound closure may contribute to postanesthetic hypothermia. Sequelae to recovery hypothermia include delayed biotransformation of anesthetic, cardiac instability, ventricular arrhythmia predisposition, CNS depression, and drug potentiation.

Prevention of hypothermia by warming fluids and using circulating warming pads and esophageal-probe monitors in the operating room is important, but this cannot always be achieved. Once the animal is in recovery, controlled warming without pulling heat from the body core to the periphery and the prevention of thermal injury are paramount. Circulating warm-water blankets and warm blankets serve this purpose well.

MALIGNANT HYPERTHERMIA

Malignant hyperthermia is a heritable muscle-disorder response to anesthesia occurring most commonly in humans and in pigs [27,28]. It also has been reported in the dog, the cat, the horse, and wild animals. The genetic factors contributing to potentially lethal changes in the skeletal muscle physiology are not well understood. An animal may have a heritable predisposition but not undergo a crisis of malignant hyperthermia, because triggering mechanisms such as stress also play a role in the disorder. Other such environmental factors include trauma, pain, and the specific anesthetics encountered. Halothane and succinylcholine have long been implicated as triggers. Malignant hyperthermia may occur in response to any anesthetic agent, however, as well as postanesthetically when the agent is cleared.

Early detection of malignant hyperthermia is critical. The earliest clinical sign in one study was an increase in ET_{CO_2} levels [27]. These values markedly increased within 10 minutes of halothane administration in some cases. Clinical signs to follow are unstable blood pressure, tachycardia, skin mottling, tachypnea, limb rigidity, changes in the electrocardiogram consistent with hyperkalemia, and myocardial hypoxia. Peak rectal temperatures developed at 35 to 60 minutes after induction in the study cited [27].

Treatment should be viewed from a perspective of crisis intervention and aggressive management. Hyperventilation with 100% O_2 and removal from anesthetic is the primary step. Dantrolene should be offered at 1 mg/kg until effect [4]. Some clinicians place a ceiling of 10 mg/kg on the dose, but it was found to be safe at 100 mg every 5 minutes in one study of dogs [4]. Bicarbonate should be given at 1 to 2 mEq/kg increments until acidosis is corrected, and cool physiologic saline should be offered intravenously. Lidocaine may contribute to hyperthermia; and arrhythmias should be treated with procainamide [28]. Assuming recovery, the animal should be watched for renal failure and a minimum urine output of 2 mL/kg/h maintained [28]. Dantrolene is recommended postanesthically to prevent relapse. Recurrence within 8 to 10 hours after recovery is not uncommon, and one case of a malignant hyperthermia crisis occurring 24 hours postanesthetically has been reported in the greyhound [28].

REFERENCES

1. Cohen MM, et al: A survey of 112,00 anesthetics at one teaching hospital (1975–1983). *Can Anesth Soc J* 33:22–31, 1986.
2. Muir WW, Hubell JAE: *Handbook of veterinary anesthesia*. St. Louis, 1989, Mosby–Year Book.
3. *Metofane® Inhalation Anesthetic*. Pitman Moore: Washington Crossing, NJ.
4. Paddleford RR: *Manual of small animal anesthesia*. New York, 1988, Churchill Livingstone.
5. Warren RG: *Animal health technology—small animal anesthesia*. St. Louis, 1983, Mosby–Year Book.
6. Short CE: *Practical use of the ultrashort-acting barbiturates*. Princeton Junction, 1983, Veterinary Learning Systems.
7. Short CE: Dissociative anesthesia. In Short CE, ed. *Principles and practice of veterinary anesthesia*. Baltimore, 1987, Williams & Wilkins.

8. Dodman NH: Pathophysiological changes of the hepatic system. In Short CE, ed. *Principles and practice of veterinary anesthesia*. Baltimore, 1987, Williams & Wilkins.
9. Paddleford RR: Anesthetic waste gases and your health. In Short CE, ed. *Principles and practice of veterinary anesthesia*. Baltimore, 1987, Williams & Wilkins.
10. Milligan JE, Sablan JL: Waste anesthetic gas concentrations in a veterinary recovery room. *J Am Vet Med Assoc*, 181:1540–1541, 1982.
11. Manley SV, McDonell WN: Anesthetic pollution and disease. *J Am Vet Med Assoc*, 176: 515–518, 1980.
12. Brodsky JB: Exposure to anesthetic gases: a controversy. *Assoc Oper Room Nurses* 38: 132–141, 1983.
13. Abraham E: Immunologic mechanisms underlying sepsis in the critically ill surgical patient. *Surg Clin North Am* 65:991–1000, 1985.
14. Wingfield WE: Cardiopulmonary arrest and resuscitation. In Etttinger SJ, ed. *Textbook of veterinary internal medicine*. Philadelphia, 1989, WB Saunders.
15. Morgan RV: *Manual of small animal emergencies*. New York, 1985, Churchill Livingstone.
16. Jacobs G: Cyanosis. In Ettinger SJ, ed. *Textbook of veterinary internal medicine*. Philadelphia, 1989, WB Saunders.
17. Davenport HW: *The ABC's of acid–base chemistry*. Chicago, 1974, University of Chicago Press.
18. Bedford PGC: *Small animal anesthesia: the increased risk patient*. London, 1991, Bailliere Tindall.
19. Webb AI: Postoperative care and oxygen therapy. In Short CE, ed. *Principles and practice of veterinary anesthesia*. Baltimore, 1987, Williams & Wilkins.
20. Hendricks JC: Respiratory conditions in critical patients. *Vet Clin North Am* 19: 1167–1188, 1989.
21. Edwards LM: Transtracheal catheterization for oxygen therapy. *Vet Tech* 9:26–32, 1988.
22. Haskins SC: Monitoring the critically ill patient. *Vet Clin North Am* 19:1059–1077, 1989.
23. *The SARA TRANScap ETCO2 Monitor®*. PPG Biomedical Systems, August 1989.
24. Short CE: Anesthetic considerations in the canine and feline. In Short CE, ed. *Principles and practice of veterinary anesthesia*. Baltimore, 1987, Williams & Wilkins.
25. Tams TR: Vomiting, regurgitation and dysphagia. In Ettinger SJ, ed. *Textbook of veterinary internal medicine*. Philadelphia, 1989, WB Saunders.
26. Harvey RC, Short CE: The use of isoflurane for safe anesthesia in animals with traumatic myocarditis or other myocardial sensitivity. *Canine Pract* 10:18–23, 1983.
27. Nelson TE: Malignant hyperthermia in dogs. *J Am Vet Med Assoc*, 198:989–994, 1991.
28. Kirmayer AH, Klide AM, Purvance JE: Malignant hyperthermia in a dog: case report and review of the syndrome. *J Am Vet Med Assoc*, 185:978–982, 1984.

9

Communication

ROBIN McGEHEE, BA, CVT

It is impossible to place too high a premium on quality communication. While a standard of excellent communication can be the life blood of any business, its value is inestimable in a hospital setting, where life-and-death decisions must be made with complete understanding by all of the parties involved. Communication with clients also can be especially challenging in situations supercharged by the emotional nature surrounding a decision to relegate a pet to surgery, coupled with what often seems to be an exorbitant amount of money.

Communication between staff members is critical to the well-being of the patient as well as the smooth operation of the hospital or clinic. Whether the staff conducts itself as a team can make or break the ongoing success of the hospital. Failure by staff members to convey information to one another after surgery can render a procedure worthless, no matter how successful that surgery might have been initially.

Lastly, communication with our patients serves as an integral component in their recovery and sense of well-being. A kind word or gentle caress often can do what no medication or sophisticated monitoring equipment can, which is to provide assurance to the animal that is often bewildered, confused, and in varying degrees of discomfort.

Communication with clients, patients, and other staff members is challenging in the critical-care setting. In all cases, emphasis must be placed on clarity and precise delineation of the facts, coupled with compassion and concern for those involved.

CLIENTS

The hospital setting presents a frightening specter for many people. Previous bad experiences or confusion about the patient's status and prognosis can leave a client feeling unsure about their ability to make the appropriate decisions regarding their animal's further care and treatment. It is up to the clinician to explain the patient's status, prognosis, and treatment options clearly and succinctly. There should be no gray areas in the client's mind. Explication of the facts must be made in a firm but compassionate manner, especially in situations where the prognosis is poor. In cases of elective surgery, one hopes that the attending clinician has underlined the potential risks and complications associated with the procedure before surgery and that no surprises will occur with which the client needs to cope. In the emergent situation, however, it is particularly incumbent on the clinician to explain the necessity for surgery to the client's satisfaction, listen to the client's concerns, give as realistic a prognosis as possible, and keep the client informed regarding changes in the patient's status.

Because there are no absolutes in terms of prognosis, recovery time, surgical odds, or expense, clients frequently are left feeling as though the decisions they make are little more than a gamble based on the educated opinion of someone whom they likely have never met. This frequently renders the decision-making process an agonizingly slow one, which compounds the frustration of everyone involved, especially when the animal must suffer the consequences. Under no circumstances, however, must the client be made to feel that he or she has been forced into making a hasty decision regarding the patient's treatment. The client must be comfortable with the explanation of the animal's physical compromise and completely understand the treatment options available to them as well as the approximate costs of those treatments. Failure to allow a client time to sort through information regarding their pet's physical status, to accustom themselves to the idea that their pet may not live despite the best efforts of the hospital staff, to accept that no matter whether the animal lives or dies they will be held responsible for the cost of treatment, and to deal with the often overwhelming emotions inherent in this situation is to open the door to a host of potential problems as the situation unfolds. Not the least of these problems is an accusation by the client that because they were not allowed ample time to consider their options, they are not liable for costs incurred because their decision-making abilities were impaired and the decision made under duress. Worse still is the situation in which the client believes their pet was subjected to treatment that resulted in wrongful death because they were not fully informed, despite the best efforts of the clinician to do so.

All of these actions and reactions are defense mechanisms enacted by people who feel frightened, guilty, and helpless in a situation they cannot fully comprehend nor fully decide regarding the health and well-being of a family member. It is up to the entire hospital staff, from the clinician to the receptionist, to recognize these defense mechanisms for what they are and remain supportive and compassionate. This should be done no matter how difficult the client may become, unless the client is so combative, abusive, or unrealistic in their expectations that it is impossible to obtain their consent for treatment given the unforseeable complications that exist in even the most minor trauma or surgical case.

There are many ways to enhance the comfort level of the traumatized client in the emergency-room setting, but excellent organization on the part of the clinician coupled with a strong support staff are a must. When four, five, or more cases are waiting in the emergency room to be seen, the ability to effectively triage cases is invaluable. It seems obvious that cases should be seen on a per-need basis rather than as first come, first served. There are clients, however, who will not understand why their pet is not attended to immediately when the animal's paw is bleeding from a laceration. These clients must be addressed pleasantly and with concern, and they should be helped to understand that they have not been forgotten and that the attending clinician will be with them shortly. They must not be lightly dismissed with "Oh, it's just a cut pad." Rather, the staff's concern must be felt by the client to be as great for this animal and client as for the client whose pet has been hit by a car and suffered massive internal injuries. If the client believes from the outset that the staff cares about their needs and those of their pet as much as they do, it will set the needed tenor of communication from the outset and quickly institute a feeling of trust by the client for the hospital and staff. In an ideal world, each patient would be assessed on arrival, treatment briefly elucidated, and the noncritical patients left by the owner to receive treatment as time allowed or the client and patient left to consider treatment options in a private exam room while other cases are similarly handled. Because the emergency room setting is far from ideal, it is important to initiate and maintain good client relations from the outset, no matter how great the tension or stress associated with the case. As veterinarians and technicians, we are responsible not only for treating sick and injured animals but for helping their human companions through what often can be one of the most traumatic events of their lives.

When difficult decisions must be rendered, the staff should try to share information and prognosis with the client so that they can make an informed decision. Owners deeply appreciate frank, candid information given on a timely basis. It is important to remember that it is their decision, and once made, it must be respected. Avoid the trap of "what you would do if it were your animal" by giving them the information they need to make the decision. One should avoid appearing condescending or superior, and mix caring and compassion within any client discussion. Also, once the decision to euthanize has been made, it is strongly suggested that a client consent form be signed and logged into the file, and that the euthanasia be carried out immediately by the clinician or other qualified personnel.

When death occurs and the client must be informed, it is desirable to do it in person whenever possible. It is important to state clearly and simply that their animal has died. A simple statement that their pet is dead is preferable to saying, for example, "We lost Rex." Or, "Rex has passed on," or some other similar euphemistic statement. You should indicate your concern for them, but do not apologize for their animal's demise. It may be appropriate to contact the owner after several hours to make cremation arrangements or ask permission for necropsy. It also is appropriate to send a note of sympathy or, if the hospital has the capability, to send a memorial gift.

STAFF

As mentioned in the introduction to this chapter, outstanding communication between staff members is essential to the success of the hospital. The larger the staff, the greater the need to facilitate clear, concise communication. It is simply unacceptable to say, "I told Sally to tell you that the surgery was rescheduled and that you were to notify the owners." Or, "Who was supposed to tell the night staff that this patient needed a catheter placed for an AM surgery?" Or, "Why does the receptionist insist on paging me when I'm in surgery?" Each of these examples is the direct manifestation of poor communication, and the net result is poor client contact, inadequate preparation, and frustration with other staff members exacerbated by the already hectic pace of any full-service hospital facility.

On paper, the solutions to these problems seem relatively simple and straightforward. In reality, however, because of the complexities of human nature and the variety of personalities, strengths and weaknesses, levels of education, and the prevailing introverted nature of veterinarians and technicians, they are far from being simple or easily managed. The following are a few guidelines that may help to enhance quality communication between staff members:

1. Make requests of one another in a courteous fashion. Do not sacrifice another's feelings because you are pressed for time, despondent over a case, or flustered by a client or other staff member.

2. Do not ask other people to relay messages for you if you are at all able to deliver the message yourself.

3. Implement time for staff meetings where communication can proceed without interruption by phones, clients, or emergencies.

4. If the staff is large, it might be advisable to institute a mediator position, who can resolve interstaff quarrels without disrupting the flow of the hospital routine or involving the entire staff.

5. Do not allow an unpleasant situation to escalate. Try to deal with any problem as it arises rather than assuming it will "go away."

6. Sexual harrassment will not be tolerated from or by either gender.

7. Never worry alone. When concerned about a patient's progress or response, immediately inform others. There is no concern too insignificant that it does not warrant attention by other staff members. Often, subtle changes can be death's harbinger, and prompt recognition can be life-saving.

8. Double-check all drug dosages, and with critical drugs, make sure that those involved are aware of all potential problems. Potassium chloride, for example, is frequently added to intravenous fluids and must be adequately mixed and never given as an intravenous bolus.

9. At shift changes, make sure that verbal and written orders are stated for every patient.

10. Never assume that someone else has done something for your patient. Check carefully for special needs when the animal presents from the operating room. For example, a chest tube may need periodic suctioning, or drug therapy started in the OR may need to be continued.

11. When problems occur, quietly summon help. It is extremely important to have assigned roles for emergency situations. Staff in the recovery area should know where critical items are kept, how to use them, and how to retrieve them expeditiously.

The recovery area often is a busy place, with animals recovering from anesthesia, others in critical condition, and not infrequently, death occurring. It is vital that sound foundations exist for interpersonal staff communication.

A detailed written record for drugs administered, physiologic trends, and the patient's response should be present in the recovery area. Verbal communication is essential as new cases are presented and recovered patients are moved into the general ward. Quiet, informative dialogue is preferable to excited epithets, and this helps to enhance the quiet, efficient environment.

PATIENTS

In a busy, full-service hospital, it is possible in the effort to "get the job done" to forget the needs of the individual patient. Before drawing blood, weighing the animal, or performing any other clinical tests, an effort should be made to "make friends" with the animal, speak reassuringly, and make it as comfortable as possible in what can be a startling and anxiety-ridden situation. Similar overtures also should be made before any procedure is begun. Not only can this calm and relax the animal, thus lessening making the need for restraint, it can make an impression on the animal that will last a lifetime.

It is important to recognize that many animals will not urinate or defecate in their kennel. If at all possible, every animal that is hospitalized should be taken outside every few hours and allowed to urinate or defecate. Not only does this keep the patients physically comfortable, it is good for their mental health as well.

Finally, an effort should be made to communicate with and treat each patient as an individual. Our clients trust us to love their pets as they do, and even the most technologically advanced medical facility in the world is mediocre if it is not staffed with compassionate and caring personnel.

10

Blood Transfusion

JANET KING, BS, CVT

Blood transfusions can be essential for survival during hematologic emergencies in the postoperative patient. Indications for blood transfusions fall into three basic categories: anemias, coagulopathies, and hypoproteinemias. Therapeutic goals from the transfusion of blood or blood products include restoration of oxygen-carrying capacity, volume replacement, protein replacement, and administration of coagulation factors and platelets. Before deciding on the need for and type of transfusion, one should look at clinical signs in conjunction with the laboratory findings. Clinical signs associated with the need for a transfusion include:

A poor response to shock therapy [1–3].
Dyspnea,
Ecchymosis,
Epistaxis,
Hematuria,
Melena,
Oozing of blood (from a venipuncture or surgical incision),
Pale mucous membranes,
Petechiation,
Prolonged capillary-refill time,
Tachycardia, and
Tachypnea.

A drop in the packed cell volume (PCV) should not be the only guideline used when deciding whether a transfusion is indicated. This is especially true in the hemorrhaging patient. Assessment of the PCV during the first 8 to 12 hours after hemorrhage is not accurate, because dilution of erythrocytes from fluid pulled into the vascular space may not have occurred [4]. Also, an animal's PCV may decrease by 10% with the administration of shock doses of fluids [3]. As a general rule, if the PCV falls acutely to 20%, a transfusion will probably benefit the patient [3]. In patients with chronic anemia, transfusion to prevent hypoxia may be required if the PCV falls below 15% in the dog and 12% in the cat [4]. When assessing the animal after transfusion, it also is important to remember that the full effect of the transfusion may not be realized for 12 to 24 hours after its completion [5]. It is important to be aware that the O_2 demand of a postoperative patient may increase 20% to 50% above baseline, so surgical drops in the PCV may double or quadruple the cardiac output in an effort to compensate [6]. Additionally, myocardial oxygenation is inadequate if the PCV is acutely lowered [7].

Because there are variable reasons for giving a transfusion, it follows that the type of transfusion required in these instances also will vary. There is a growing trend in veterinary medicine regarding use of blood-component therapy. Use of components is more economical, because one donation can help more than one animal. Component therapy can improve the results of treatment by replacing only what the animal needs, thereby decreasing the chance of circulatory overload. In addition, use of components reduces the number of transfusion reactions by exposing the animal to fewer antigens [3]. With use of a refrigerated centrifuge, a unit of whole blood can be processed into components such as packed red blood cells (RBCs), plasma (fresh and frozen), platelet-rich plasma, and cryoprecipitate (a product of fresh-frozen plasma). The most commonly used components are packed RBC and fresh frozen plasma. These components can be made without the use of a refrigerated centrifuge by allowing a unit of whole blood to separate naturally under refrigeration ($1°$ to $6°$ C) for 18–24 hours, however the plasma will have reduced clotting factors.

WHOLE BLOOD

Whole blood contains all cellular and plasma components. Indications for a whole-blood transfusion include sudden, massive hemorrhage as a result of surgery or trauma, or a coagulopathy with active bleeding [8]. An acute loss of 30% to 40% of blood volume results in hypovolemic shock. Fresh whole blood also can be used in the patient requiring clotting factors and/or platelets if transfused within 6 hours of collection. If platelets are required, the whole blood should not be refrigerated.

PACKED RED BLOOD CELLS

Usually, the hematocrit of packed RBCs is approximately 80% [3]. Compared with whole blood, packed cells contain less citrate and fewer foreign proteins and antigens, which may decrease the possibility of a transfusion reaction [9]. This component is required when an animal needs increased O_2-carrying capacity. There is no advantage to using stored whole blood over packed RBCs as a treatment of acute hemorrhage [10]. Hemorrhagic shock can be treated with crystalloid and colloid solutions followed by a packed RBC transfusion [10]. Packed RBCs also are indicated in chronic anemias, where the animal has a decreased PCV with normal plasma-protein values [2]. If the patient is at risk of fluid volume overload, packed RBCs are a better choice over whole blood [2,8]. Packed RBCs also have been shown to increase plasma volume by causing the movement of fluid and albumin from the extravascular space into the circulation [9,10]. Movement of albumin into the capillaries can replace up to 50% of lost blood volume without the need for supplemental plasma [10]. Therefore, a transfusion of packed RBCs can increase the plasma volume to the same degree as 2 to 3 U of plasma [9].

PLASMA

Plasma is a source of hemostatic proteins (factors and cofactors of the clotting cascade, von Willebrand's factor), albumin, and globulin.

Fresh Plasma

Fresh plasma is separated from RBCs within 3 to 4 hours and is used within 24 hours [11]. Fresh plasma contains all coagulation factors and plasma proteins such as albumin and globulins [12,13].

Fresh-Frozen Plasma

Fresh-frozen plasma is separated and frozen to $-30°$ C within 6 hours of collection and has an expiration date of 1 year from collection [10,13]. It contains coagulation factors and plasma proteins [12,13].

Frozen Plasma

Frozen plasma is plasma that has been frozen for between 1 and 5 years, or plasma that has been separated and frozen after more than 6 hours from the time of collection [10,11]. Frozen plasma has reduced levels of factors VIII and V, but it will contain the stable, vitamin K–dependent factors II, VII, IX, and X [10]. Frozen plasma also is a source of albumin and globulin.

Cryoprecipitate Plasma

Cryoprecipitate is prepared by thawing fresh-frozen plasma at 4° C [11]. The cold-precipitated material is a concentrated source of factor VIII, von Willebrand's factor, fibrinogen, and fibronectin [10]. Cryoprecipitate is used primarily to treat hemophilia A and von Willebrand's disease [10].

Coagulation Factors and Plasma Proteins

Albumin is difficult to supply intravenously in adequate amounts to reverse hypo-albuminemia. When assessing the degree of hypoalbuminemia, the total albumin deficit (both intravascular and extravascular) must be considered; therefore, the volume of plasma required to correct the deficit is large [9]. The concentration of albumin in 1 U of plasma is approximately 3 g/dL, and the amount of plasma that can be administered at one time will probably increase the albumin in the recipient by only 1 g/dL [3]. A transfusion of plasma for the replacement of protein may be indicated if the hypoproteinemia is reversible, as would occur in bacterial pleuritis or peritonitis with repeated drainage of effusion, parvovirus in young puppies, and acute hepatic necrosis where hepatic regeneration would restore normal protein values [3]. A transfusion of plasma may be beneficial if the serum albumin falls acutely to 1.5 g/dL or the total protein is less than 5 g/dL [2,8]. In puppies, plasma may be required if the total protein is less than 3.5 g/dL [2]. If albumin is being lost via the kidneys or the gastrointestinal tract, any albumin administered through a transfusion also would be lost [10]. Sixty percent of total albumin is located in the interstitial spaces and would move into the intravascular space to increase plasma albumin; therefore, hypoproteinemia may be better treated by parenteral or enteral alimentation [9,10].

Plasma also can be used as a source of antibodies for passive immunity. A transfusion of plasma can provide antibodies to orphaned puppies and kittens and for other viral diseases, such as parvovirus in dogs [14].

Replacement of active clotting factors requires a transfusion of fresh plasma, fresh-frozen plasma, or cryoprecipitate [3]. If these products are unavailable or RBCs also are required, fresh whole blood can be used. Some of the more common reasons for a transfusion with plasma are hemophilia A (factor VIII deficiency), hemophilia B (factor IX deficiency), von Willebrand's disease (deficiency of von Willebrand's factor, a protein necessary for normal platelet function), and acquired coagulation disorders such as those occuring with liver disease, vitamin K deficiency, and disseminated intravascular coagulation (DIC) [3]. DIC is commonly associated with hemangiosarcoma and other malignancies, immune-mediated hemolytic anemia, gastric torsion, pancreatitis, heat stroke, liver disease, and infection [10] Fresh or fresh-frozen plasma can be used as a source of coagulation proteins in the treatment of DIC, and also as a source of antithrombin III, which can help to prevent further thrombosis associated with DIC [10].

PLATELETS

Platelet-rich plasma is separated from whole blood by centrifuging at a slower speed at room temperature. Platelet-rich plasma contains approximately 75% of the platelets found in the same volume of whole blood [3].

Clinical signs of thrombocytopenia usually are not evident until the platelet count drops below 50,000/μL [3]. Clinical signs associated with a deficiency of platelets include petechiation of skin and mucous membranes as well as bleeding of mucosal surfaces [3]. Transfused platelets have a relatively short half-life, usually lasting from a few hours to, at most, 72 hours [1,3]. Animals requiring platelets usually require repeated transfusions over several days. These animals then run the risk of immune sensitization to the platelets and white blood cells [15]. If severe thrombocytopenia with active bleeding results from a metobolic disorder or drug therapy, the animal may benefit from a transfusion of platelets until the underlying problem can be corrected [3]. If thrombocytopenia is immune-mediated, the transfused platelets will quickly be destroyed. Both the short half-life of platelets and the method of preparation and storage makes use of platelet-rich plasma undesirable in veterinary medicine. Fresh whole blood can be used to supply platelets and should be kept at room temperature and transfused within 6 hours [3].

AUTOTRANSFUSION

Autotransfusion can be life-saving in cases of severe hemorrhage when a rapid transfusion is necessary and donor blood is unavailable. The procedure involves the collection of autologous blood from an active bleeding site in the pleural or peritoneal cavity and its reinfusion back into the patient's circulation. Research has shown that survival time of the reinfused erythrocytes is no different when compared with that of normal cells [16]. Because an animal is receiving its own blood back, isoimmunization to erythrocytes, leukocytes, platelets, and other protein antigens does not occur. This fact makes autotransfusion a useful alternative in situations where excessive bleeding is encountered rather than relying on multiple transfusions of donor blood [16]. Also, the patient is assured of receiving warm, fresh, compatible blood.

Autotransfusion is not without risk. Complications include hemolysis, coagulation disorders, microembolism, sepsis, and tumor metastasis (if blood contains neoplastic cells) [17]. Hemolysis can occur when a suction device is used to salvage the blood, especially if a large amount of turbulance and foaming occurs because of high negative pressure [16,17]. Care should be taken not to combine air with blood during suctioning, because air triggers hemolysis [18]. The transfusion of a large number of hemolyzed RBCs can initiate DIC [17]. Adequate volume replacement usually will prevent complications resulting from hemoglobinemia [16,17].

Other complications of autotransfusion are coagulation disorders. Platelet aggregation and subsequent thrombocytopenia can occur when blood comes in contact with air or serosal surfaces [16,17]. Also, activation of the coagulation mechanism can occur with the initiation of DIC [16,17]. Thrombocytopenia is a normal occurance of extracorporeal bypass, including autotransfusion. Studies have shown that platelet counts never decrease below $50,000/\mu L$ during autotransfusion [16].

Microembolization is another complication following autotransfusion; however, the extent to which it occurs is unknown [17]. It generally is recommended that blood be filtered before reinfusion into a patient. Use of a $40\text{-}\mu m$ filter will remove the majority of micoaggregates, although in most situations, a standard $170\text{-}\mu m$ filter may suffice [19]. Corticosteroids (e.g., prednisolone, 30 mg/kg body weight) administered during autotransfusion have been shown to protect lungs from the effects of lung embolism [18]. Microaggregates also release substances such as serotonin, histamine, kinens, and catecholamines [16]. These vasoactive substances cause bronchoconstriction, increased pulmonary vascular resistance, and pulmonary hypertension [16,17].

Autotransfusion is contraindicated in cases of malignancy or if the blood to be reinfused has been contaminated with bile, fat, urine, or feces [16–18]. In life-threatening situations, however, the benefit of autotransfusion may outweigh the risk of using blood contaminated with urine, bile, or fecal material [18]. Blood that has been in contact with pleural or peritoneal surfaces for over 24 hours should not be used for autotransfusion [16]. Prolonged contact of blood to serosal surfaces causes in increased number of microaggregates, severe hemolysis, and higher incidence coagulation defects [16].

Collection of blood from the pleural cavity or the peritoneum can be performed using either a simple system of syringes and suction or a commercial autotransfusion unit (Solcotrans Autologous Whole Blood Transfusion System, Solco Basle, Rockland, Mass.) (Fig. 10–1). Blood that has been in contact with serosal surfaces longer than 45 minutes will not clot; therefore, anticoagulant is not necessary [19]. If a transfusion is necessary immediately on hemorrhage, gentle suction can be used to aspirate the blood into a 60-mL syringe containing 9 mL of acid, citrate, dextrose anticoagulant (ACD) [19]. The blood should be filtered before reinfusion. A Hemonate Filter (Gesco International, San Antonio, Tex), (Fig. 10–2) can be attached between the syringe and intravenous line. Commercially available blood-collection sets using a vacuum bottle containing ACD and a standard blood filter also can be used [16].

A heparin-flushed, 60-mL syringe and a system involving a four-way stopcock

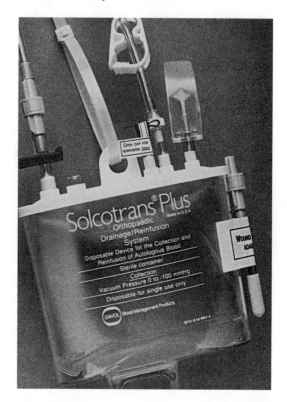

Fig. 10–1. Example of autologous blood-collection and reinfusion container/systems.

and intravenous tubing has been successful in small animals (Fig. 10–3) [16]. By manipulating the syringe and four-way stopcock, blood can be aspirated from a closed hemothorax or hemoperitoneum. This technique also can be used when the thorax or abdomen is open in surgery (Fig. 10–4) [16].

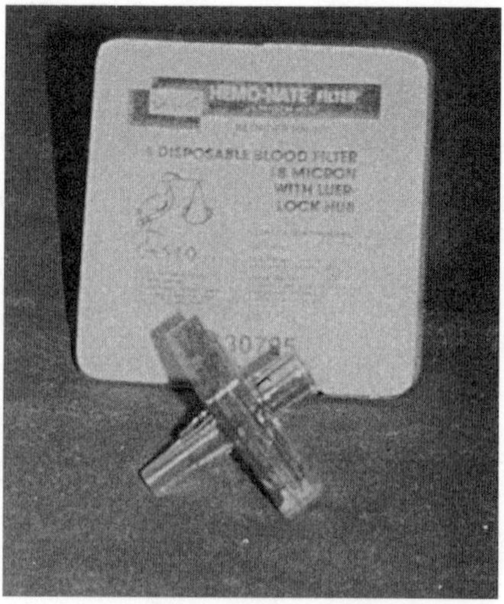

Fig. 10–2. Hemonate filter used for the transfusion of small amounts of blood from a syringe.

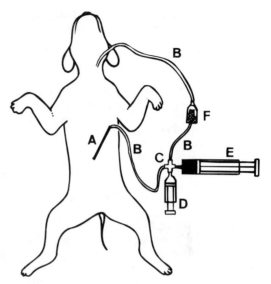

Fig. 10–3. Autotransfusion in a small dog in which blood is being aspirated from the abdominal cavity. Note the peritoneal dialysis catheter (*A*), intravenous extension tubing (*B*), four-way stopcock (*C*), 3-mL syringe containing heparin (*D*), 60-mL syringe (*E*), and micropore transfusion filter (*F*). (With permission from D.T. Crowe, Jr., D.V.M. Autotransfusion in the trauma patient Veterinary Clinics of N. America Vol. 10 no. 3 Aug 1980 p. 583–584, W.B. Saunders.)

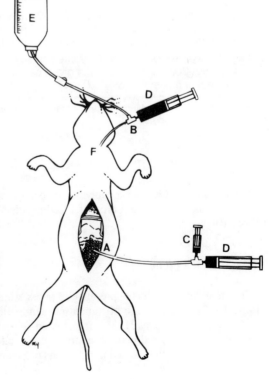

Fig. 10–4. Autotransfusion during surgery in a cat. Note the gauze sponge with the tip of the intravenous extension tubing inside the abdominal cavity (*A*), three-way stopcock (*B*), 3-mL syringe containing heparin (*C*), 60-mL syringe (*D*), balanced salt solution (*E*), and jugular catheter (*F*). A peritoneal dialysis catheter (not shown) may be used as a suction tip to allow easier aspiration of the blood. (With permission from D.T. Crowe, Jr., D.V.M. Autotransfusion in the trauma patient Veterinary Clinics of N. America Vol. 10 no. 3 Aug 1980 p. 583–584, W.B. Saunders.)

Table 10–1
Dosages for Blood and Blood Products

Dosages for whole blood and packed RBC
1. 2.2 mL/kg (1.0 mL/lb) of whole blood will increase the recipient's hematocrit by 1% if the donor's hematocrit is 40% if a dog and 30% if a cat.
1.0 mL/kg of packed RBCs will increase the recipient's hematocrit by 1% if the hematocrit of the packed red cells is 80%.
2. $$\text{Dose of anticoagulated whole blood} = \frac{\text{recipient blood volume} \times \text{desired PCV} - \text{actual PCV of recipient}}{\text{PCV of donor blood}}$$
88 mL/kg (dog)
66 mL/kg (cat)

Dosages for plasma
1. For hypoproteinemia: 6–10 mL/kg.
2. For active bleeding because of coagulation protein deficiency:
   a. 6–10 mL/kg 2–3 times a day until active bleeding stops.
   b. 1 u of plasma per 10–20 kg – measure pre- and post-PT and APTT. If transfusing prior to surgery, give 1 hr. before anesthesia
3. For passive immunity: 1 mL/oz body weight of puppy to a maximum of 10 mL, then 3–5 mL thereafter. Repeat as needed daily or 1–2 times per week.

Dosages for platelets:
1. Dosage of whole blood to increase platelets (use fresh whole unrefrigerated blood within 6 hours): 250 mL of fresh whole blood with a platelet count of 200,000/μL will increase the platelet count of a 20-kg dog by approximately 13,000/μl.
2. Dosage for platelet-rich plasma: Platelet-rich plasma extracted from 500 mL of whole blood will increase the platelet count of a 30-kg dog by approximately 10,000/μL. Or give 3–5 mL/lb once or twice daily.

Dosage for cryoprecipitate: 1 u of cryoprecipitate (formed from 1 u of plasma, approximately 150–200 mL of plasma) is given per 10 kg of body weight every 8 hours until bleeding has stopped.

APTT = Activated partial thromboplastin time; PCV = packed cell volume; PT = prothrombin time; RBC = red blood cell.

DOSAGES OF BLOOD AND BLOOD PRODUCTS

The volume of blood or components to be administered will depend on the degree of anemia, the severity and type of bleeding disorder, and the size of the animal (Table 10–1).

ADMINISTRATION

Crossmatching detects the presence of preexisting antibodies against erythrocytes (Table 10–2). The half-life of transfused, compatible RBCs is 20 days in the dog and 30 days in the cat [3]. The transfusion of incompatible RBCs decreases the survival time of the red cells to approximately one third that in autologous RBC transfusions [5]. With repeated transfusions of incompatible blood, the survival time decreases even more.

Table 10–2
Cross-Match Chart

---

1. Recipient samples:
   a. Collect 2 mL of recipient blood into a serum tube and 1–2 mL of recipient blood into an EDTA or heparin tube.
   b. Separate the serum and plasma from the red blood cells by centrifugation.
2. Donor Samples:
   a. Collect 2 mL of donor blood into a serum tube and 1–2 mL of donor blood into an EDTA or heparin tube.
   b. Separate the serum and plasma from the red blood cells by centrifugation.
   c. Alternatively, remove one or two segments of tubing from the donor blood bag and gently mix the contents of the tube. Collect 2 mL of the donor blood into an empty tube. (This blood already contains anticoagulant.) Separate the plasma from the red blood cells by centrifugation.
3. Wash the two tubes of packed red blood cells (obtained from anticoagulated blood) as follows:
   a. Add 2–3 mL of 9% saline to each tube and resuspend the red blood cells.
   b. Centrifuge the tubes and discard the supernatant.
   c. Repeat this procedure two more times.
4. Prepare a 4% red-blood-cell suspension of donor and recipient red blood cells. A 4% suspension can be made by mixing 0.2 mL of packed red blood cells with 4.8 mL of 9% saline.
5. Set up four tubes as follows:
   a. Donor control: two drops of donor plasma or serum and one drop of donor 4% red-blood-cell suspension
   b. Recipient control: two drops recipient serum and one drop of recipient 4% red-blood-cell suspension
   c. Major cross-match: two drops of recipient serum and one drop of donor 4% red-blood-cell suspension
   d. Minor crossmatch: two drops of donor plasma or serum and one drop of recipient 4% red-blood-cell suspension
6. Ideally the three sets of the tubes listed in step 5 should be set up for incubation at different temperatures:
   a. Incubate one set for 15 minutes at 4°C.
   b. Incubate one set for 15 minutes at room temperature (25°C).
   c. Incubate one set for 15 minutes at 3°C.
   d. If unable to set up tubes at all three temperatures, perform the crossmatch at 25°C and 37°C.
7. Following incubation, centrifuge all tubes and examine the supernatant for hemolysis. Gently tap the tubes to resuspend the red cells and observe for agglutination. The control tubes should not react. The major and minor crossmatch tubes should be compared with the control tubes.
8. The presence of agglutination of hemolysis in the major or minor crossmatch indicates an incompatible crossmatch. It is strongly recommended that a different donor be used.

EDTA = Ethylenediaminetetraacetic acid.

The major crossmatch (donor's RBCs and recipient's serum) is the most clinically significant, because it detects recipient antibodies to donor cells [3]. The minor crossmatch (donor's serum and recipient's RBCs) detects antibodies in the donor's serum against the recipient's cells. Dogs do not have significant naturally occuring antibodies against erythrocyte antigens; therefore, an initial crossmatch on a dog that has not been transfused or pregnant should be compatible [21]. An exception to this would be a dog with autoimmune hemolytic anemia. Cats with type-B blood do have strong naturally occuring antibodies (anti-A); therefore a crossmatch would detect an AB mismatch [21]. Ideally, donor and recipient blood should be cross-matched before each transfusion. Cross-matching may not be possible in all situations (e.g., emergencies, lack of staff) but should be performed if the donor animals are not typed, the recipient has had previous transfusions or multiple transfusions are forseen, or if transfusing a cat [1,2]. Plasma can be transfused without concern for blood type, because few RBCs are present and the donor plasma should not have preexisting antibodies [10].

BLOOD ADMINISTRATION

Blood and blood components should be shaken gently and warmed to room temperature. Rapid administration of cold blood can cause hypothermia and cardiac arrhythmias [11]. The blood bag can be immersed in a warm-water bath (37° to 38° C) (Fig. 10–5) [12]. It generally is recommended that blood and blood products be

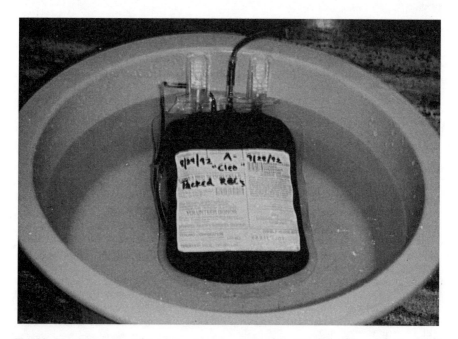

Fig. 10–5. Warm-water bath used to slowly warm blood and blood products to room temperature.

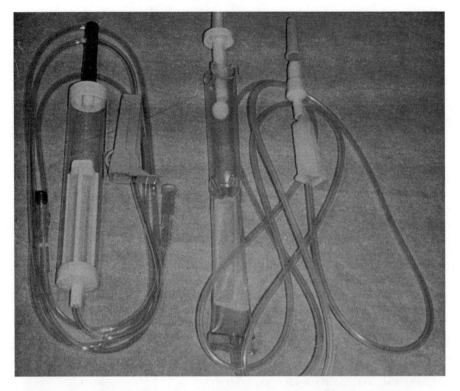

Fig. 10–6. Blood filters used for the transfusion of blood and blood products.

administered through a filter to trap blood clots and other debris (Fig. 10–6). Most standard blood-administration sets contain a 170-μm filter. For administering small amounts of blood from a syringe (e.g., transfusion in a cat), a Hemonate Filter (Gesco International, San Antonio, Tex.) can be used [13].

Other important guidelines for the storage and handling of blood include:

1. Blood is an excellent medium for bacterial growth. If blood is kept out of the refrigerator for longer than 30 minutes, transfuse within 6 hours or return it to the refrigerator and reduce the expiration date to 24 hours from the time it left the refrigerator [13].
2. Once fresh-frozen plasma has thawed to room temperature, transfuse immediately or delete the word ''fresh,'' return it to the refrigerator, and reduce the expiration date to 24 hours from the time it left the refrigerator. If thawed in the refrigerator, plasma can be refrozen as frozen plasma, but its shelf-life should be cut in half [13].
3. Do not freeze whole blood or packed RBCs.
4. Platelets are not viable in refrigerated or frozen products.

Isotonic saline (0.9%) is the only fluid/drug that should be administered in conjunction with blood. Lactated Ringer's solution, dextrose solutions, and hypotonic saline never should be administered with blood through the same intravenous line [11]. The citrate anticoagulant binds calcium, and the calcium present in lactated Ringer's solution may cause coagulation [11]. Dextrose solutions may cause agglutination, hemolysis, or both [4,11].

The preferred route of administration for blood and blood products is intravenously through a catheter. Intraosseous is a useful route for small puppies and kittens. Absorption of blood via the intraosseous route is rapid, at a rate of approximately 1 drop per second [22]. The intraperitoneal route is the least favorable. Blood absorption is slow (i.e., only 40% after 24 hours) and the RBCs have a shortened life span [12].

The rate of administration depends on the hydration status, degree of anemia, and general health of the animal. Before beginning a transfusion, baseline values of temperature, pulse, respiratory rate, mucous membrane color, PCV, and total protein should be recorded [11]. The maximum rate in a well-hydrated animal is 10 mL/lb/h, although a dehydrated animal may be able to withstand a rate of 30 mL/lb/h [21]. In an animal with heart failure, the rate should not exceed 2 mL/lb/h [21]. Syringe replacement in small animals should be given at 1 mL/min [5]. Plasma administration should occur over a 2- to 4-hour period [10]. The transfusion should be given slowly for the first 20 to 30 minutes to observe for a possible transfusion reaction [2,11]. If no problems appear in the recipient, the transfusion rate can be increased. Platelet-rich plasma should be given slowly, because platelet fragments and released histamine or serotonin can cause shivering, salivation, urticaria, and restlessness [15].

RESPONSE TO BLOOD TRANSFUSIONS

It is important to closely monitor the recipient of a blood transfusion both during and after the procedure. An animal receiving a transfusion of RBCs should show improvement in mucous membrane color, capillary refill time, pulse quality, respiratory rate, and patient strength [3] within hours of the transfusion. Hematocrit and total protein should be measured 2 to 4 hours after the transfusion and then at frequent intervals [2,3]. Because of the equilibration of fluid, the actual posttransfusion PCV may not be evident for 12 to 24 hours following the transfusion [22].

The effectiveness of coagulation proteins supplied by a plasma transfusion can be shown by cessation of blood loss and increase in the PCV [3]. Laboratory measures of clotting times also can be used to guage the effectiveness of the plasma transfusion [3]. Platelet counts can be done to measure increases in the number of platelets.

ADVERSE TRANSFUSION REACTIONS

Adverse transfusion reactions can result from incompatibility between donor and recipient as well as improper collection, storage, and administration. With the exception of cats with type-B blood, transfusion reactions in veterinary medicine are rare because of the low levels of naturally occuring isoantibodies in animals. Transfusion reactions can be classified as either immune mediated and nonimmune mediated. Immune-mediated reactions consist of acute hemolytic reactions; delayed hemolytic reactions; adverse reactions to leukocytes, platelets and proteins; and neonatal isoerythrocytolysis [11]. The severity of these incompatibility reactions will vary with the titer of circulating isoantibodies in the recipient and the amount of incompatible blood transfused. Delayed hemolytic reactions are more common than acute hemolytic reactions. Delayed reactions can be subclinical and not noticeable. In a delayed transfusion reaction, the survival time of the RBCs is shortened, and there may be an unexpected drop in the PCV [11,23].

An acute hemolytic reaction occurs because the recipient has preformed antibodies to the donor blood, resulting in intravascular hemolysis [14]. Acute hemolytic reactions result in fever, vomiting, collapse, hypotension, tachycardia, hypopnea, pigmenturia, neurologic signs, shock, and DIC [3,5,21,23]. These signs can appear within seconds of the infusion of incompatible blood [21]. Dogs rarely will have an acute reaction following the first transfusion of incompatible blood because of their low levels of naturally occuring isoantibodies [23]; however, the recipient will produce isoantibodies that will shorten the half-life of the transfused erythrocytes to approximately 7 to 10 days [24]. Acute hemolytic reactions can occur in dogs previously sensitized by a prior transfusion and in cats with type-B blood given type-A blood [3]. Blood type–B cats have strong, naturally occuring anti-A antibodies, so the incompatible RBCs would survive only minutes to hours, and the transfusion would cause serious clinical signs [14]. If signs of an acute hemolytic reaction occur, the transfusion should be discontinued immediately. Treatment should be instituted to maintain blood pressure and renal blood flow and to prevent DIC [23]. Controversy exists as to whether immune-mediated hemolytic reactions can be prevented or lessened by pretreating the recipient with antihistamines or steroids. It is best to avoid the possibility of an immune-mediated hemolytic reaction by blood-typing donors, crossmatching, and administering only compatible blood.

Nonimmune-mediated hemolytic transfusion reactions can occur when blood is hemolyzed before the transfusion. This can occur with improper storage and handling of blood. Blood can become hemolyzed by overheating or freezing, mixing the blood with hypotonic solutions, contamination with hemolytic bacteria, and mechanical trauma to the RBCs during drawing or administration [23]. These problems can be prevented by proper handling and by using appropriate techniques.

The most common clinical sign associated with a transfusion reaction is fever, followed by vomiting [21]. Vomiting can occur because of too-rapid administration of blood [22]. Most febrile reactions are mild and result from the donor's leukocytes and sensitization of the recipient to the donor's histocompatibility antigens [21,23]. If the animal only develops a fever, the transfusion can be continued and antipyretics administered when the temperature exceeds 104° F [21]. Fever in the recipient also can occur with bacterial contamination of the blood. If the blood is contaminated, the reaction is immediate and severe, and it is usually accompanied by trembling, acute collapse, endotoxic shock, and possibly, DIC [5,23]. If this occurs, the transfusion should be discontinued and the remaining untransfused blood Gram stained. The animal should be treated for shock and started on intravenous antibiotics [23].

Allergic reactions are rare but have been seen in both canine and human patients [23]. Allergic reactions in the recipient occur because of foreign antigens in the donor plasma and result in urticaria and edema [23]. If the allergic reaction is severe, the transfusion should be discontinued and the animal given antihistamies and possibly epinephrine [23]. If the allergic reaction is mild, the recipient can be given an antihistamine and the transfusion continued at a slower rate [11,23].

Circulatory overload is most likely to occur in small, normovolemic animals and in those with cardiac disease [23]. Chronically anemic animals are at greater risk of circulatory overload because of cardiac hypertrophy or dilatation occuring from increased cardiac output [23]. Signs of circulatory overload include cough, cyanosis, dyspnea, and moist rales caused by pulmonary edema [5,23]. The risk of circulatory overload can be minimized by using packed RBCs and by monitoring the central venous pressure [5,11,23]. If circulatory overload is suspected, the transfusion should be discontinued and the animal treated with diuretics and O_2 [5,23].

Citrate is metabolized rapidly by the liver, so citrate intoxication is rare. Citrate intoxication may occur, however, with rapid, multiple transfusions or in animals with severe liver disease, portosystemic shunts, or hypothermia [5,23]. Components with the most citrate are fresh-frozen plasma, platelet-rich plasma, and whole blood [23]. An overdose of citrate can cause electrocardiographic abnormalities, muscle tremors, hypotension, and hypocalcemia [5,11,23]. If citrate intoxication is suspected, the transfusion should be stopped for 5 to 10 minutes and then restarted at a slower rate [23]. Intravenous calcium gluconate also can be given if necessary [5,11,23].

The transfusion of cold blood can result in hypothermia in the recipient. This is especially important in the postoperative patient with anesthetic-induced hypothermia. If the body-core temperature decreases to 30° C, ventricular dysrrhythmias and cardiac arrest can occur [5]. Warming the blood before a transfusion will minimize hypothermia [11].

Transmission of infectious agents through a blood transfusion has been well documented in humans. The transmission of retroviruses through infusion of contaminated blood is important in cats, cattle, and horses [23]. Five percent of cats have been shown to carry either the feline leukemia virus or the feline immunodeficiency virus [23]. *Hemobartonella felis* also has been shown to be transmitted via a blood transfusion [1,23]. Depending on geographic location, dogs may be at risk for transfusion-transmitted babesiosis, ehrlichiosis, Rocky Mountain spotted fever, brucellosis, borreliosis, and the microfilarial stage of dirofilariasis [1,23]. The transmission of disease through a transfusion can be minimized by testing the blood to be transfused as accurately as possible for the presence of infectious agents.

REFERENCES

1. Crystal MA, Cotter SM: Acute hemorrhage: a hematologic emergency in dogs. *Comp Cont Ed Pract Vet* 14:60–67, 1992.
2. Oakley DA, Shaffran N: Blood transfusions. Part II. Collection, storage, and administration. *Vet Tech* 8:189–193, 1987.
3. Brooks M: Transfusion medicine. In Murtaugh RJ, Kaplan PM, eds. *Veterinary emergency and critical care medicine*. St. Louis; 1992, Mosby–Year Book, pp. 536–546.
4. Pichler ME, Turnwald GH: Blood transfusion in the dog and cat. Part I. Physiology, collection, storage, and indications for whole blood therapy. *Comp Cont Ed Pract Vet* 7:64–71, 1985.
5. Raffe MR: Intravenous therapy and blood transfusion. In Bright RM, ed. *Surgical emergencies*. New York; 1986, Churchill Livingstone, pp. 25–36.
6. Gump FE, et al: Oxygen consumption and caloric expenditure in surgical patients. In Slatter D, ed. *Textbook of small animal surgery*. Philadelphia, 1993, WB Saunders, pp. 212–224.

7. Cloves GHA Jr, et al: The cardiac output in response to surgical trauma. *Arch Surg* 81: 212–222, 1960.
8. Killingsworth CR: Blood banking for the feline and canine patient. *J Vet Crit Care* 7: 1–10, 1984.
9. Stone E, Badner D, Cotter SM: Trends in transfusion medicine in dogs at a veterinary school clinic: 315 cases (1986–1989). *J Am Vet Med Assoc* 200:1000–1004, 1992.
10. Cotter SM: Rational use of plasma. In *Proceedings of the 59th annual meeting.* New Orleans, 1992, American Animal Hospital Association, pp. 74–77, April 25–30, 1992.
11. Authement JM, Wolfsheimer KJ, Catchings S: Canine blood component therapy: product preparation, storage, and administration. *JAAHA* 23:483–493, 1987.
12. Turnwald GH, Pichler ME: Blood transfusion in dogs and cats. Part II. Administration, adverse effects, and component therapy. *Comp Cont Ed Pract Vet* 7:115–124, 1985.
13. Carlin S: *Blood banking for every hospital.* Dixon, CA, Animal Blood Bank.
14. Smith CA: Transfusion medicine: the challenge of practical use. *J Am Vet Med Assoc* 5:747–752, 1991.
15. Dodds J: *Hemopet.* 17672-A Cowan, Suite 300 Irvine, CA 92714.
16. Crowe DT: Autotransfusion in the trauma patient. *Vet Clin North Am* 10:581–597, 1980.
17. Zenoble RD, Stone EA: Autotransfusion in the dog. *J Am Vet Med Assoc* 172:1411–1414, 1978.
18. Niebauer GW: Autotransfusion for intraoperative blood salvage: a new technique. *Comp Cont Ed Pract Vet* 13:1105–1118, 1991.
19. Gibbons G: Respiratory medicine. In Murtaugh RJ, Kaplan PM, eds. *Veterinary emergency and critical care medicine.* St. Louis, 1992, Mosby–Year Book, pp. 403–404.
20. Feldman BF, Thomason KF: Useful indexes, formulas and ratios in veterinary laboratory diagnostics. *Comp Cont Ed Pract Vet* 11:174–175, 1989.
21. Giger U: Transfusion therapy for veterinary technicians. Veterinary Technician Proceedings, 1992. North American Veterinary Conference. pp. 33–34.
22. Norsworthy GD: Clinical aspects of feline blood transfusions. *Comp Cont Ed Pract Vet* 14:469–475, 1992.
23. Cotter SM: Adverse effects of transfusions. In *Proceedings of the 59th annual meeting.* New Orleans, April 25–30, 1992, American Animal Hospital Association, pp. 78–81.
24. O'Neill S: Blood transfusions. Part I. The blood donor colony. *Vet Tech* 8:87–89, 1987.

//

Procedures and Specific Protocols

This section lists and describes the most commonly performed operative procedures. In addition, the most frequent postoperative problems associated with each procedure are catalogued. This section can be useful to the recovery team, because it can serve as a quick reference briefly describing the procedure and common postoperative problems that may occur. One must be cautious, however, because problems other than those listed may occur and present a threat to life. Only the most frequently performed procedures are listed, so it is quite probable that procedures will be performed that are not described in the text. It is incumbent on the recovery team to discuss the procedure with the surgeon and to become aware of the potential complications associated with the procedure. Using the recovery record, these potential problems can be listed to increase the awareness for all concerned with the patient's recovery. It must be understood that the common postoperative problems of hemorrhage, adverse anesthetic reactions, hypothermia, hypotension, pulmonary embolism, infection, and others may occur in association with the procedures listed in the following section.

11

Neurosurgical Procedures

Patients recovering from neurosurgery often have special postoperative demands. These animals may have various levels of paresis or plegia and require attentive postoperative care. In the case of preexisting trauma, there may be some damage to the central nervous system. For example, a dog injured by an automobile may have both skull and vertebral fractures. Many animals undergoing neurosurgical procedures have received corticosteroids, and colonic perforation or rupture following neurosurgery has been reported [1]. In most cases, dexamethasone was used and perforations occurred in the descending colon. Colonic perforation results in rapid formation of peritonitis. Signs of shock and/or peritonitis such as hypoglycemia, hypotension, poor tissue perfusion, abdominal pain and distension, and fever present. Abdominocentesis is the diagnostic method of choice. Once recognized, treatment requires immediate repair of the perforation, removal of peritoneal contaminants, broad-spectrum (i.e., anaerobic/aerobic) antibiotics, and aggressive supportive care. The prognosis for recovery is grim.

SPINAL SURGERY

Surgery is performed on the vertebral column to alleviate lesions that are compressive to the spinal cord from disc, bone, or tumor. At times, it may be undertaken for diagnostic reasons. Unstable spinal fractures may require decompression and fracture immobilization.

DORSAL LAMINECTOMY

Dorsal laminectomy involves removing the dorsal spinous processes and the dorsal or lateral lamina of the vertebra to provide access to and decompression of the spinal cord. A laminectomy may be performed over one or several vertebral segments (Fig. 11–1).

Common postoperative problems include:

1. Pain. In spite of altered nerve transmission, laminectomy patients are subject to significant postoperative pain (see Chapter VI).

125

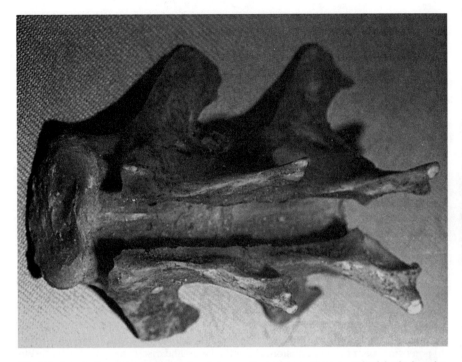

Fig. 11–1. A dorsal laminectomy has been performed over three vertebral body lengths. This procedure provides significant spinal cord decompression. (Courtesy of David M. Ennis, DVM.)

2. Hemorrhage. Incisional or subcutaneous hemorrhage, while not life threatening, can be problematic and lead to seroma formation or infection. In this procedure, hemorrhage is revealed by firm swelling associated with the incisional area that will enlarge over time. The application of ice packs and pressure wraps may help to control hemorrhage. In breeds known to harbor the von Willebrand's gene, a coagulation profile or buccal mucosal bleeding time should be done preoperatively.

3. Many patients subjected to laminectomy are paretic or plegic before surgery. These existing conditions also need care postoperatively. The animal needs to be placed on a well-padded surface (Figs. 11–2 and 11–3) to prevent decubital ulcers and turned frequently. Bladder care is mandatory to prevent urine soiling and infection. Paraparetic or paraplegic animals should be confined to a small area and not be allowed to drag themselves about (Fig. 11–4).

4. The patient's neurologic condition must be monitored carefully. For example, an animal that was paraparetic presurgically and has become paraplegic postsurgically is showing symptoms of neurologic deterioration. This deterioration may indicate ascending hematomalacia or progressive neurologic damage.

5. Bladder care. Patients with significant neurologic compromise with paresis or plegia require bladder care. The bladder should be gently expressed every 4 to 6 hours and/or catheterized if necessary. Incomplete voiding and the trauma associated with repeated expression or catheterization increase the incidence of bacterial cystitis. Antibiotics are used for specific treatment, not prophylaxis, in these cases.

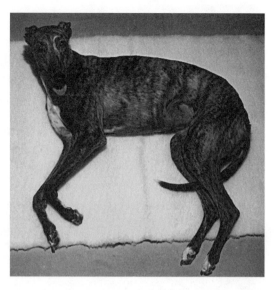

Fig. 11–2. Synthetic fleece material can be used to provide padding for paralyzed animals. As it becomes soiled, the material can be washed and reused. (Courtesy of David M. Ennis, DVM.)

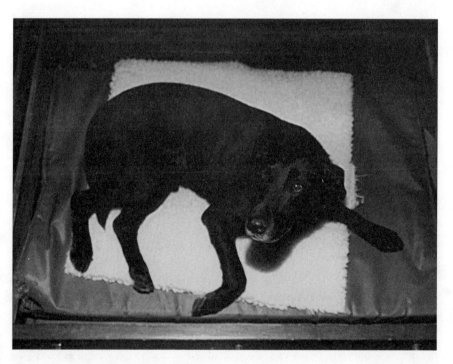

Fig. 11–3. A specially made waterbed can provide an ideal surface for a paralyzed animal. It is important to prevent urine scalding, because urine tends to pool in areas of the plastic. (Courtesy of David M. Ennis, DVM.)

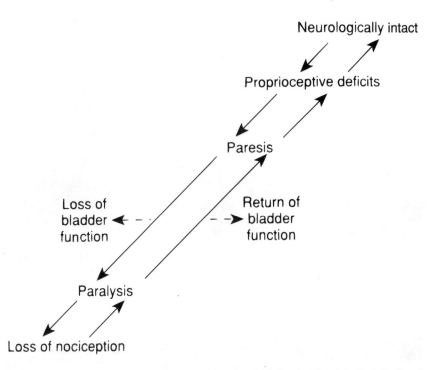

Fig. 11–4. Cascade of the loss and return of function associated with pelvic-limb dysfunction caused by spinal cord injury. A recovering animal, with return of motor function, should have urinary continence; if not, a problem such as urinary cystitis should be ruled out. (From Slatter D.E. (ed.) In: Textbook of Small Animal Surgery. Philadelphia, W.B. Saunders, pp. 563, 1993.)

6. Wound complications. Wound complications such as seromas, hematomas, infection, and dehiscence have been reported, with complication rates listed as 14% [2]. Many patients who receive laminectomies are given corticosteroids and nonsteroidal, anti-inflammatory drugs, and they are subjected to longer hospital stays and lengthy surgical procedures, all of which may contribute to the higher rate of wound complications.

HEMILAMINECTOMY

Hemilaminectomy is a form of abbreviated laminectomy that involves removal of the articular process and part of the vertebral lamina on one side (Fig. 11–5). It is performed to provide spinal decompression and allow access to the herniated intervertebral disc on either the right or left side. Hemilaminectomy allows better access to ventral or lateral compressive masses and provides direct access to ventral or lateral compressive masses and provides direct access to the ventral aspect of the spinal canal. In general, the same concerns exist for this procedure as for laminectomy.

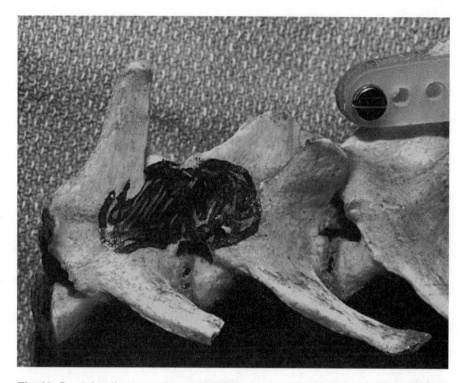

Fig. 11–5. A hemilaminectomy provides limited access to the spinal cord, but it is easier to accomplish than a dorsal laminectomy. (Courtesy of David M. Ennis, DVM.)

VENTRAL DECOMPRESSION

This procedure involves approaching the cervical vertebrae ventrally and removing a portion of the disc and vertebral body to allow access to the spinal canal and cord (Fig. 11–6). Cervical intervertebral disc disease is common in the dog and accounts for 16% of intervertebral disc problems [3]. Chondrodystrophic and other small breeds account for the majority of cases, but it also is common in larger breeds such as the Doberman pinscher. Cervical intervertebral disc disease may produce hyperpathia, ataxia, paresis, or paralysis. Patients with cervical disc disease producing nonambulatory tetraparesis are surgical and management challenges, with a perioperative mortality rate of 57% reported [3]. Complications associated with corticosteroid usage, such as melena and gastrointestinal ulceration, frequently are observed, as are decubital ulcers and urinary tract infections. This procedure is done to decompress the cervical spinal cord, remove herniated disc material, and visualize the ventral portions of the spinal cord and canal.

Common postoperative problems include:

1. Pain. This procedure involves extensive soft-tissue retraction and destruction of bone, and it is associated with significant postsurgical pain. Appropriate pain management is important to enhance a safe, nonstressful recovery (see Chapter VI).

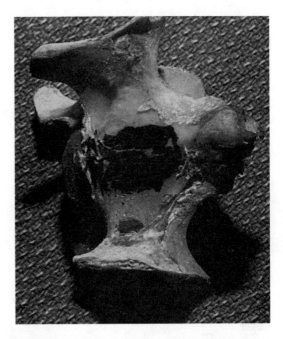

Fig. 11–6. A ventral slot procedure is performed to gain access to the ventral aspect of the cervical spinal cord and intervertebral discs. (Courtesy of David M. Ennis, DVM.)

2. Hemorrhage. The venous sinuses diverge laterally over the intervertebral disc, and the slot is made through this area. Frequently, the thin-walled venous sinuses are damaged, and significant hemorrhage occurs. Hopefully, the hemorrhage has been controlled in the operating room, but on presentation to the recovery area, the animal may have sustained significant blood loss and be hypovolemic. These animals may need volume replacement, whole blood, or packed red blood cells (see Chapter X). In some cases, airway compromise may occur, from hemorrhage resulting in the development of a hematoma in the cervical region. This can be an insidious problem that develops after extubation, and cervical radiographs or ultrasonography may be required to detect the presence of a cervical hematoma.

3. Nerve damage. The recurrent laryngeal and vagus nerves are subject to injury during the surgical approach. During the postoperative period, the patient should be observed for signs of laryngeal paralysis and Horner's syndrome (i.e., mydriatic pupils, ptosis, prominent nictitating membrane).

4. Bladder care. Many animals with cervical myelopathy are unable to adequately control bladder function. This deficit must be acknowledged and a plan formulated for periodic bladder expression and urinary care. These animals are at risk for urinary tract infection. Frequent urinalysis is appropriate.

SPINAL FRACTURES

A variety of treatment methods are used to stabilize spinal fractures, and not infrequently, a laminectomy is done for spinal decompression. Current stabilization methods include external fixation, pins, methylmethacrylate, screws, wires, and plates. Many problems associated with the neurologically compromised animal also apply to these patients.

When an external fixateur is present, it must be covered to prevent it from being caught on cage doors or other structures. While infrequent, it is possible that the fixateur will be dislodged during a violent anesthetic recovery. It also obviously is important not to allow the animal to chew on or bite the fixation device.

DISC FENESTRATION

Fenestration involves creating a window in the annulus fibrosa to allow removal and decompression of the pulpy nucleus of the disc. Cervical fenestrations usually are approached ventrally, while thoracolumbar discs are approached laterally. This procedure involves deep-muscle dissection and retraction, so excessive hemorrhage and moderate postoperative pain may be present.

INTRACRANIAL SURGERY

Intracranial procedures are done less frequently, but they often require exacting postoperative care. Intracranial surgery is most frequently performed for tumor removal, diagnosis, and/or to provide decompression. In a recent report of 31 craniotomies performed on the dog and the cat [4], the 81% survival rate indicates that the procedure is safe in experienced hands. Survival after surgery depends on the type and severity of the intracranial disease.

Increased Intracranial Pressure

With some operative procedures, or as a result of trauma, an increase in the intracranial pressure may occur. Signals of this might include tachycardia and pupillary constriction. When this occurs, appropriate drug therapy, including phenobarbitol, corticosteroids, and diuretics, is indicated. Volatile anesthetics can increase cerebral blood flow and may block autoregulation. Retention of carbon dioxide influenced by respiratory depression also may cause increased intracranial pressure. Cerebral blood flow may increase 200% with the volatile anesthetic halothane [5]. To minimize increases in intracranial pressure following surgery, good postoperative support of ventilation is needed. Avoid drugs that are potent respiratory depressants (e.g., oxymorphone); also avoid dissociatives, halothane, and nitrous oxide. It is preferable to use injectible barbiturate induction and isoflurane for maintenance anesthesia.

Dementia

Depending on the extent of the procedure, dementia or altered mental status producing a violent recovery may occur. Tranquilization or sedation may be necessary.

Coma

After intracranial surgery, animals may have a delayed recovery and present to the recovery area in a comalike state. Extra-vigilant monitoring of important physiologic parameters such as blood pressure, heart rate, temperature, and level of consciousness is mandatory.

Postoperative Neurologic Scale

The postoperative neurologic scale contains four levels:

1. Alert: normal to verbal and mechanical stimuli,
2. Lethargic: arousal can be maintained by verbal or mechanical stimulation,
3. Obtunded: requires constant mechanical stimulation to maintain arousal, and
4. Comatose: does not respond to verbal or mechanical stimulation.

Unequal Pupil Sizes

Anisocoria following cranial surgery or trauma usually means that edema or an existing mass effect has stretched cranial nerve III on the ipsilateral side. If the

Table 11–1
Neurosurgical Procedures

	Pupil Size	Reactivity	Prognosis
	Normal (midrange)	Normal	Good
	Bilateral miosis	Poor to nonresponsive	Guarded (variable, depending on other signs)
	Unilateral mydriasis	Poor to nonresponsive (mydriatic side)	Guarded to poor
	Unilateral mydriasis with ventrolateral strabismus	Poor to nonresponsive (mydriatic side)	Guarded to poor
	Normal (midrange)	Nonresponsive	Poor to grave
	Bilateral mydriasis	Poor to nonresponsive	Poor to grave

(From Dewey, et al: The Compendium North American Edition, Small Animal. (14)2;1992, p. 199).

larger pupil is reactive, then Horner's syndrome (miosis, ptosis, and prolapsed third eyelid) exists.

Pinpoint pupils in a comatose patient indicate significant higher-brain compression or injury. Fixed and dilated pupils signify massive lower-brainstem injury (Table 11–1).

SURGERY OF THE PERIPHERAL NERVOUS SYSTEM

This surgery is undertaken to explore peripheral nerves, repair trauma-damaged nerves, or less frequently, sever a peripheral nerve. In cases of nerve repair or reconstruction, it is important to protect the wound from the animal during the recovery process. Usually, the site is protected with a soft, padded bandage for 7 to 10 days. Limb immobilization with a splint or cast might be necessary if moderate tension is present across the repair.

REFERENCES

1. Toombs JP, et al: Colonic perforation in corticosteroid treated dogs. *J Am Vet Med Assoc* 188:145–150, 1986.
2. Hosgood G: Wound complications following thoracolumbar laminectomy in the dog. A retrospective study of 264 procedures. *JAAHA* 28:47–52, 1992.
3. Toombs JP: Cervical intervertebral disc disease in dogs. *Compend Cont Ed Pract Vet* 14: 1477–1489, 1992.
4. Niebauer GW, et al: Evaluation of craniotomy in dogs and cats. *J Am Vet Med Assoc* 198: 89–95, 1991.
5. Van Poznak A: Special considerations for veterinary neuroanesthesia. In Short CE, editor: *Principles and Practice of Veterinary Anesthesia*. Baltimore, 1987, Williams & Wilkins.

12

Surgery of the Alimentary Tract

LIPS AND CHEEKS

Surgery involving these structures can include repair after trauma, tumor excision, or reconstructive surgery. It is important after surgery to prevent self-mutilation and airway obstruction from blood or mucus.

TONGUE

Tongue surgery usually involves repair of traumatic lacerations or infrequent tumor excisions. Dogs and cats rarely swallow their tongues. The pharynx must be cleared of any blood or mucus. Tongue lacerations are painful, and the animal may have difficulty eating or lapping water postoperatively. The canine/feline tongue is very vascular, and significant blood loss can occur with major lacerations. In some cases of severe hemorrhage from tongue lacerations, the animal may need whole blood, packed red blood cells, or volume replacement.

The authors have observed animals presented to the emergency room with significant tongue lacerations and severe hypovolemic shock. On presentation, however, there is little evidence of hemorrhage, as the animal swallows most of the blood and the resulting hypotension reduces blood flow from the laceration.

DENTAL PROCEDURES

Dental extractions may ooze after surgery, but in the hemostatically healthy patient, this rarely is a problem. Dental reconstructions, complex gingivectomies, and endontia must be protected. One must ensure that the animal does not bite or chew on the cage bars, and the animal may require a soft, moist diet or gruel for several days after surgery. Excessive hemorrhage following dental extractions may indicate a pre-existing coagulopathy.

CLEFT RECONSTRUCTIONS

Once a cleft-reconstructive surgery has been accomplished, the pharynx should be cleared of mucus and blood. In the case of soft-palate resection, one should open the mouth periodically and examine the surgical site for excessive hemorrhage.

PHARYNGOSTOMY

Pharyngostomy usually is done to place a tube from the pharyngeal region to the distal esophagus through a stab incision in the pharyngeal region. Placement of a pharyngostomy tube should avoid the adjacent vascular structures, and the skin and pharynx should be inspected for signs of hemorrhage. The tube should be secured with tape, suture, and bandage material to prevent accidental removal or dislodgment. In many cases, an Elizabethan collar will be necessary to prevent the animal from pawing at the tube. The pharyngostomy tube should be closed securely with either a cap or a clamp to prevent gravitational leakage of the stomach contents. This procedure has been replaced by tube gastrostomies or enteral feeding methods.

TONSILLECTOMY

Tonsillectomy is increasingly rare in the dog and cat. It involves excision and suture ligation of the tonsillar bed. Alternatively, one may electrocoagulate the bleeding vessels of the tonsillar bed.

Hemorrhage can be problematic after a tonsillectomy and may produce airway obstruction and aspiration. Animals should be observed carefully for evidence of oral hemorrhage, coughing, or choking as an indication of obstruction.

FRACTURES OF THE MAXILLA/MANDIBLE

Fractures of the maxilla and mandible may be repaired with many techniques. These include external fixation, pins, wires, and screws. They also may be managed with tape muzzles (Fig. 12–1).

After any oral procedure, one must check for airway obstruction from blood or mucus. In some instances, the jaws may be immobilized with wire and make clearing the airway more problematic. It also is important that the patient not be allowed to paw or otherwise dislodge external fixateurs or acrylic splints.

SALIVARY GLANDS

In a recent review of pathology records [1], diseases of the salivary glands accounted for 3% of all cases. Thirty percent of the reported cases were malignant (i.e., adenocarcinoma or carcinoma), 26% were diagnosed as sialadenitis, and 16% were judged to be normal salivary tissue [1].

Surgery of the salivary glands most commonly involves removal of one or more glands because of the formation of a salivary mucocele. The common duct of the mandibular and sublingual salivary glands becomes obstructed or ruptures, and saliva accumulates in the cervical and submandibular area. Neoplasia of the salivary glands may be treated with wide surgical excision in an effort to obtain surgical margins free of tumor.

Many surgeons will place a drain in the wound bed and mucocele. It is important to protect this drain from displacement. Other, less frequently reported postsurgical complications include damage to the jugular veins, damage to the facial nerves, perforation of the pharynx, and abscess formation.

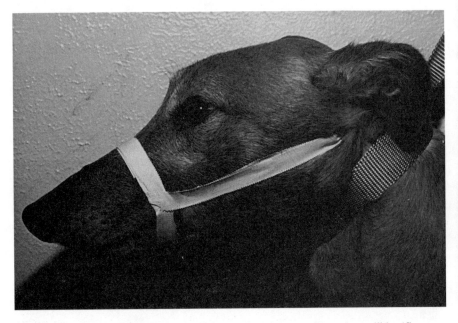

Fig. 12–1. A tape bridle used to stabilize fractures of the maxilla and mandible. (Courtesy of David M. Ennis, DVM.)

SALIVARY GLAND NEOPLASIA

As previously mentioned, adenomas and carcinomas of the salivary glands do occur, with the parotid gland being the most commonly involved. Often, surgical removal and the need for tumor-free margins of normal tissue create large dead-space defects that necessitate placement of some form of wound-bed drainage.

ESOPHAGUS

Esophageal surgery may be done to remove foreign bodies, excise neoplastic lesions, repair lacerations or perforations, or correct vascular-ring abnormalities or to reduce gastroesophageal intussusception. A thoracostomy is required for intrathoracic esophageal surgery, and thoracostomy management is covered in Chapter VII. With some severe perforations or lacerations, the patient may be managed with a gastric or jejunal tube for temporary alimentation.

Gastroesophageal intussusception can be an acute, life-threatening problem. In some individuals, especially those with a history of megaesophagus, intussusception may occur during recovery. Alteration of venous return and gastric blood flow may produce shocklike signs. These animals also may salivate profusely, paw at their mouths, and have increasingly severe dyspnea. Thoracic radiographs and fiberoptic esophagoscopy are useful in diagnosing this problem (Fig. 12–2).

Once the problem is identified, the patient is stabilized and returned to the operating room for reduction and stabilization of the intussusception. Gastroesophageal

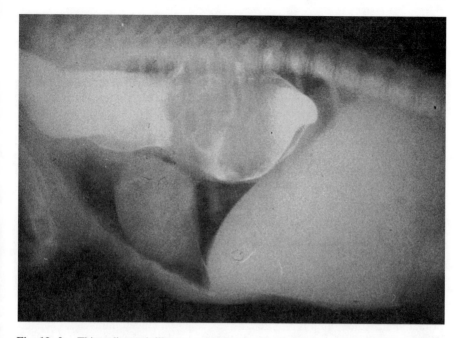

Fig. 12–2. This radiograph illustrates a soft-tissue density in the caudal esophagus, which is a gastroesophageal intussusception. (Courtesy of Norm Ackerman, DVM.)

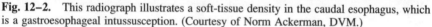

intussusception is an infrequent disease associated with preexisting megaesophagus. In 23 reported cases, 83% of patients were dead within 3 days, and a correct antemortem diagnosis was made in only 5 cases [2]. In any case involving esophageal surgery, nursing orders for food and water should be defined clearly.

ESOPHAGEAL FOREIGN BODIES

Esophageal foreign bodies are most common in small dogs (body weight, <12 kg), and a variety of objects ranging from bones to fish hooks have been encountered. Most commonly, the object can be removed via fiberoptic esophagoscopy or advanced into the stomach. The majority of foreign bodies lodge in the distal esophagus proximal to the gastroesophageal junction. Esophageal perforations occur in approximately 25% of cases [3] and are managed by either thoracotomy or laparotomy and primary repair of the perforation. Mortality rates approaching 60% have been reported [4].

In all cases of esophageal foreign bodies, complications such as esophagitis, perforation, pneumomediastinum, pneumothorax, pneumonia, pleuritis, and mediastinal and esophagobronchial fistulae may occur. Foreign bodies usually can be removed using a rigid or fiberoptic endoscope per os. Once the foreign body is removed, the esophageal mucosa can be visualized for necrosis, laceration, or perforation. Because air insufflation is common with esophagoscopy, a pneumomediastinum or pneumothorax may occur if a full-thickness esophageal laceration is present. When endoscopic retrieval of foreign bodies is unsuccessful, thoracic esophagoscopy is indicated.

Postoperative complications include:

1. Leakage or dehiscence. These problems most often occur in the days following surgery and are caused by excessive tissue necrosis from the foreign body, inadequate tissue debridement, or improper technique.

2. Infection. Perforations or extensive mucosal necrosis may allow translocation of microorganisms to occur. Broad-spectrum antibiotics are indicated when mucosal damage is present.

3. Stricture. Full-thickness, circumferential mucosal damage may produce an esophageal stricture.

Postoperative management considerations include:

1. If a thoracotomy has been performed, normal management principles for this procedure are indicated (see Chapter VII).

2. Antibiotics can be used either prophylactically or to treat existing esophageal infection.

3. Fluid and electrolyte maintenance is useful for a normal recovery. Restriction of oral alimentation often is required, necessitating prolonged intravenous support. With extensive esophageal injury, oral alimentation is restricted for 5 to 7 days. In these cases, alimentation can be supplied via a gastrostomy or jejunostomy tube.

4. Additional drug therapy. When gastroesophageal reflux is suspected, pharmacologic inhibition of gastric acid may be helpful. Cimetidine (5–10 mg/kg orally every 6 hours) or Zantac (ranitidine, Glaxo Pharmaceuticals, Research Triangle Park, N.C.; 1–2 mg/kg orally twice daily) by nature of the histamine-receptor blockade may be given. Metoclopramide (0.2 mg/kg orally three times per day with cimetidine, weight restriction, and a high-protein low-fat diet) may increase lower esophageal sphincter tone and reduce esophageal reflux.

MEGAESOPHAGUS

Megaesophagus rarely is treated surgically, but its presence should be acknowledged as it can cause postsurgical problems. Aspiration of esophageal contents, esophageal infection, or gastroesophageal intussusception are more likely in patients with existing megaesophagus.

ESOPHAGEAL NEOPLASIA

Esophageal neoplasia accounts for less than 5% of all cancer in the dog and cat [5], but often is very advanced. Surgical removal of esophageal neoplasia and repair of the resultant defects can be very challenging. The postoperative team should obtain specific orders from the surgeon in managing these patients postsurgically.

GASTRIC SURGERY

Gastric surgery commonly is performed for foreign-body retrieval, correction of gastric torsion, biopsy, obstructional relief, or excision of neoplasia. Specific postoperative concerns for each problem are discussed later.

GASTRIC DILATION AND VOLVULUS

Gastric dilation and volvulus (GDV) is a frequently seen and challenging surgical problem. Animals with GDV often present to the emergency room with severe dyspnea, gastric distension, and distress. Once a diagnosis has been made and the animal's condition temporarily stabilized, surgery is indicated. Surgery involves derotating and then stabilizing the stomach with some form of gastropexy, and it may include resection of necrotic stomach and splenectomy.

The postoperative management of GDV patients is always challenging. When possible, an established postoperative protocol will prevent omission of care and allow proactive treatment. Mortality rates of from 20% to 40% are not uncommon [6], and the interval of time before presentation, presurgical decompression, and shock stabilization are important factors influencing mortality.

Other considerations regarding postoperative care include:

1. Fluid and electrolyte maintenance. Large volumes of isotonic fluids may be used during stabilization. Frequent measurement of PCV, total solids, and Na^+ and K^+ electrolyte values can be useful. Hypokalemia is the most common electrolyte abnormality (i.e., <3.5 mEq/mL) and probably results from potassium loss and sequestration in the torsed stomach. Empiric supplementation with 20 to 40 mEq of potassium chloride per liter of intravenous fluids has been suggested [7]. There are a large number of potential postoperative complications associated with GDV syndrome and the surgery performed to correct it (Table 12–1). As this syndrome is common, the postoperative team should have a heightened awareness of these potential problems.

2. Urinary output should be monitored to ensure renal production and to avoid fluid overload. This may involve closed urinary catheterization or just routine observation of urinary output.

3. Acid–base balance may be altered after surgery, with severe metabolic acidosis present. When possible, routine measurement of arterial or venous pH is used both to treat and monitor acid–base disturbances.

4. Cardiac arrhythmias often occur postoperatively because of the release of reperfusion products. Continuous cardiac monitoring with a telemetry unit can be helpful in diagnosing and monitoring this problem. Postoperative GDV patients should routinely receive procainamide. As many as 40% to 50% of dogs develop ventricular arrhythmias after surgery [8], and Table 12–2 serves as a suggested protocol for arrhythmia control after GDV surgery. Treatment for ventricular arrhythmias is started if the frequency is greater than 15/min or if signs of altered cardiovascular function are present (i.e., decreased oxygen saturation; weak, thready pulse; poor capillary refill; unstable blood pressure; or generalized weakness).

Table 12–1

Postoperative Complications Associated with Gastric
Dilation-Volvulus Syndrome

Shock
Ventricular arrhythmias
Sepsis/endotoxemia
Reperfusion injury
Gastric necrosis/gastric rupture
Peritonitis
Anemia
Hypoproteinemia
Acid–base imbalance
Gastric atony
Pneumothorax
Disseminated intravascular coagulopathy
Gastric dilation
Incisional infection/dehiscence
Gastrectomy leakage/dehiscence
Foley catheter displacement (tube gastrostomy technique)
Bronchopneumonia/aspiration pneumonia
Pancreatitis
Pulmonary abscessation
Renal failure
Hepatopathies
Hemorrhage
Intestinal volvulus
Intestinal intussusception
Esophagitis
Gastric ulceration/gastritis
Volvulus recurrence

Table 12–2

Control of Premature Ventricular Contractions in the Patient with Gastric Dilation
and Volvulus

Lidocaine 2% solution
    1–2 mg/kg intravenous slow bolus
    Give half the amount initially, followed by the remainder slowly over 3 to 5 minutes
    May be given as continuous infusion: 1 mg/kg slow bolus followed by 10–15 μg/
    kg/min continuous infusion
    Following elimination of arrhythmia longer acting antiarrhythmic agents are used
Quinidine sulfate
    1.5–5 mg/kg every 2 hours orally until arrhythmia is controlled, then every 6 to 8
    hours
Quinidine gluconate
    1.5–5 mg/kg every 3 to 6 hours intramuscularly
Procainamide hydrochloride (regular formulation)
    Sustained-release form is poorly absorbed
    1.5–5 mg/kg orally or intramuscularly every 2 hours until arrhythmia controlled, then
    every 4 to 6 hours
    1.5–5 mg/kg loading dose intravenously over 5 minutes, followed by 2.5–9 μg/kg/
    min as continuous infusion

---

5. A complex disease, GDV may produce a plethora of postsurgical problems. These may include iatrogenic injuries, surgical complications, wound complications, or systemic responses to the disease itself. Possible problems associated with GDV are:

Iatrogenic injuries: Rib fractures
Pneumothorax
Laceration to abdominal viscera
Massive blood loss
Pancreatitis
Surgical complications: Gastric rupture/gastric dehiscence
Gastrostomy tube complications or dislodgement
Technical failure of gastropexy
Peritionitis
Wound complications: Infection
Herniation
Systemic complications: Aortic thromboembolism
Pancreatitis
Disseminated intravascular coagulation
Pneumonia
Renal failure
Myocarditis

PYLOROPLASTY

Pyloroplasty is done to enlarge the gastric outlet and therefore alleviate gastric retention. This may involve an incision through the seromuscular layer of the pyloric region or a more aggressive technique of reconstruction. This procedure usually is an elective operation.

Postoperative complications include:

1. Incisional leakage or dehiscence. The most common surgical procedure to correct pyloric stenosis involves incising the seromuscular layer of the pylorus, leaving the intact mucosa to bulge through the incision (Fig. 12–3). Provided that the mucosa is intact, leakage is an infrequent problem.

2. Hemorrhage is an infrequent problem in the hemostatically healthy patient.

3. Iatrogenic injury to the common bile duct, pancreatic duct, or pancreas. Iatrogenic injury in these locations is uncommon. Injury of this type might produce biliary obstruction or leakage and/or pancreatitis in the days following surgery.

4. Vomiting and persistent outflow obstruction. Postoperative vomiting may occur after gastric surgery. After surgical recovery, small amounts of water are offered, and if vomiting does not occur after 8 to 12 hours, the patient is offered small amounts of soft, moist food. Some surgeons use metoclopromide postoperatively for several days to reduce vomiting.

GASTRODUODENOSTOMY AND GASTROJEJUNOSTOMY

The Billroth I and Billroth II procedures (Fig. 12–4) were named for the German surgeon who developed them. In small animals, these procedures usually are done

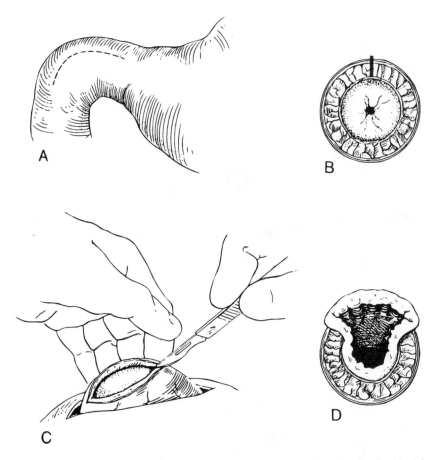

Fig. 12–3. A Fredet-Ramstedt pyloromyotomy is done by creating a longitudinal incision in the pylorus only through the seromuscular layer. The mucosa bulges through the incision. (From Slatter, D.: Textbook of Small Animal Surgery. Philadelphia, W.B. Saunders, 1993, p. 998.)

as a part of cancer resection. Billroth procedures are technically demanding and require rigorous operative technique. The alleviation of normal gastrointestinal function can produce jejunal ulcers, bloating, and intestinal ileus.

Considerations in postoperative care include:

1. Blood and fluid loss. A procedure of this magnitude often results in significant blood or fluid loss. Prompt recognition of loss and replacement thereof is critical during the postoperative period.

2. Pain management. As part of an established hospital protocol, appropriate pain management should be instituted in the operating room and continued postoperatively.

3. Jejunal intussusception. Intussusception of the jejunum into the stomach after gastrojejunostomy has been reported [99]. This problem presents a challenging post-

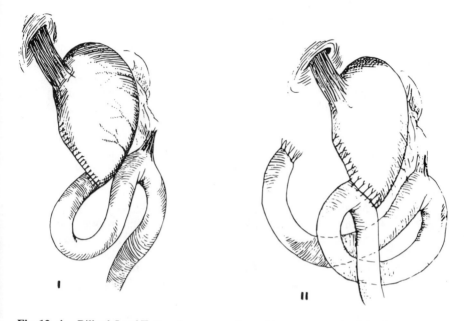

Fig. 12–4. Billroth I and II procedures are performed to remove proximal duodenal, pyloric, and gastric lesions. (From JAAHA, 25(2);1990 p. 217.)

surgical diagnosis, and radiographs and/or ultrasound are required for confirmation. Once a diagnosis has been made and the patient stabilized, reoperation is mandatory to correct the problem.

4. Anastomatic leakage and peritonitis. Anastomatic leakage and breakdown may occur at any time. Animals with leakage within the first 24 hours may be hemodynamically unstable and slower to recover from anesthesia. Signs of shock including hypotension, poor tissue perfusion, and diminished urinary output may be present. Alternatively, signs of early septic shock such as brick-red mucus membranes, tachycardia, hypoglycemia, and fever also may be present. Diagnostic abdominocentesis is performed and the aspirated fluid examined for cell type, total-solid levels, bacteria, and especially bacteria-laden neutrophils. The presence of large numbers of microorganisms in phagocytes or a vast array of gram-positive and gram-negative organisms is reliable proof that leakage has occurred.

5. Iatrogenic pancreatic or biliary tract damage has been observed.

6. In cases of gastrojejunostomy, marginal ulceration of the proximal jejunum has been reported; however, this occurs in the weeks or months following surgery [10].

GASTRIC FOREIGN BODY

When oral gastroscopy fails to retrieve a foreign body, it must be removed surgically. Following entry into the abdomen, the ventral aspect of the stomach is incised and the material removed. Following removal, the stomach wall is closed, with closure of the abdominal wall occurring next.

Postoperative concerns include:

1. Nausea and vomiting. Following gastric surgery, nausea and vomiting may occur. This usually can be controlled with metoclopromide HCL or other antiemetics and by keeping the patient NPO until the nausea and vomiting resolve.

2. Aspiration pneumonia. Aspiration is possible after pyloric outlet surgery. With pyloric obstruction, the stomach may be distended with fluid. During anesthetic relaxation of the gastroesophageal constriction, the fluid subsequently may move into the esophagus. During recovery from anesthesia, while the patient is still recumbent, the fluid is easily aspirated. When this problem is anticipated, the stomach and esophagus may be suctioned of their contents to prevent aspiration.

3. Depending on the type of foreign body and the severity and duration of vomiting, fluid and electrolyte imbalances may be present. Hopefully, these have been identified presurgically and treatment replacement will extend postoperatively. Of particular concern is metabolic alkalosis occurring with pyloric obstruction. Acid–base status and electrolyte determination should be done postoperatively if the patient's condition so warrants.

4. Small amounts of water are offered after anesthetic recovery. If the water is retained, small quantities of food (I/D Hill's Pet Products, Topeka, Kans.) may be offered 12 hours after surgery.

INTESTINAL SURGERY

Intestinal surgery is a commonly performed procedure in small animals. Both the large and small bowel may be incised, resected, and anastomosed. The breakdown of enterotomy repairs and anastomoses are the most common and devastating problems which occur. This situation invariably leads to local or generalized peritonitis, and it may result in septic shock and death. When this problem occurs in the immediate postoperative period, it is because of improper suturing technique, incorporation of devitalized bowel through loss of blood supply, or acute bacterial peritonitis resulting from surgical contamination. Abdominocentesis, as previously described, is the single best means of detecting leakage of intestinal contents into the peritoneal cavity.

INTESTINAL DEHISCENCE

Dehiscence of enterotomy or anastomotic closures occurred in nearly 16% of cases in one series [11], with a reported mortality rate of 74%. The mean time for dehiscence was 3.90 ± 1.8 days, and those patients with intestinal trauma or foreign-body entrapments had a significantly higher risk of dehiscence. In addition, males were at a greater risk for dehiscence than females.

INTUSSUSCEPTION

Intussusception results from trauma, irritation, or inflammation to the bowel, and it is caused by one segment of bowel contracting and forcing the intestine into the lining of an adjacent, relaxed segment. This problem may occur after enterotomy or anastomosis. It may be more frequent when there is severe bowel trauma or irritation. It may happen in the immediate postoperative period or in the following days.

The level of intussusception will influence the emergence and severity of clinical signs. A proximal jejunal intussusception more rapidly produces intestinal obstruction, fluid, acid–base, and electrolyte changes or abnormalities than does an ileocolic intussusception. Clinical signs, physical examination, radiographs, and ultrasonography are used to diagnose this problem. Intussusception most frequently occurs in young animals and is often a recurring problem (Fig. 12–5).

ILEUS

Ileus is an uncommon postsurgical problem in small animals. It is characterized by an adynamic small bowel occurring as a result of anesthesia and surgery. Because of its adynamic state, ileus produces a form of intestinal obstruction. It is more likely to be a problem either when peritonitis exists or subsequent to abdominal surgery. Clinically, the animal may exhibit vomiting and anorexia, and the abdomen may appear distended. Fluid- and gas-filled loops of bowel are seen radiographically, and ileus must be differentiated from generalized peritonitis. Metoclopromide

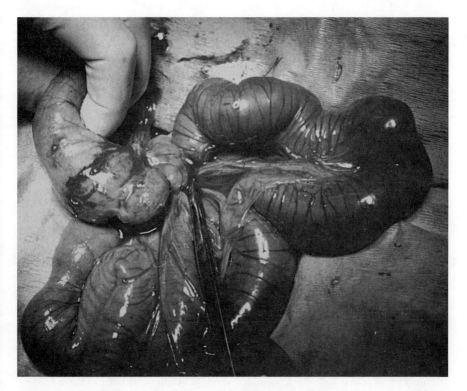

Fig. 12–5. Recurrent intussusception in a 4-month-old mixed-breed dog. (Courtesy of Peter Schwarz, DVM.)

(0.2–0.4 mg/kg intravenous or intramuscular) is given every 4 hours to stimulate intestinal motility.

EXPLORATORY LAPAROTOMY

Exploratory laparotomy is a commonly performed procedure used to treat, diagnose, or stage a variety of problems. Procedures may range from simple herniorrhaphy or abdominal-wall laceration, to complex partial hepatectomy or nephrectomy. Treatment and evaluation of abdominal trauma or neoplasia are the most common reasons to perform a laparotomy. The peritoneal cavity is invaded via one or more approaches to gain access to the structures within. The procedure performed in the abdomen will directly influence the frequency and occurrence of postoperative complications.

Elective umbilical herniorrhaphy has a very low morbidity and mortality rate, whereas herniorrhaphy associated with extensive bite wounds has a reported infection rate of 50% [12]. Exploratory celiotomy is not a benign procedure, with complication rates of 30% reported [13]. Disease-related complications are observed twice as frequently as surgical complications.

When possible, early resumption of feeding restores normal gastrointestinal reflexes and motility. The point at which one resumes oral feeding is important. In general, water is offered after recovery from anesthesia, and food is offered 12 hours later. In cases of severe peritonitis, extensive bowel trauma, or resection, nutritional support may be necessary. This may necessitate placement of a gastric or small intestine feeding tube (see Chapter IV).

LARGE BOWEL PROCEDURES

While less common, surgical procedures involving all or part of the large bowel still are performed. It often is difficult to prepare the large bowel for surgery, and there is a higher postoperative infection rate. Patients recovering from large intestinal surgery are carefully assessed for signs of peritonitis or leakage. Abdominocentesis is performed whenever warranted by clinical observation or if signs of peritonitis or leakage are present.

In cases of advanced peritonitis, the peritoneal cavity is opened surgically and maintained in that manner for several days to promote effective drainage of the entire peritoneal cavity. Sterile laparotomy sponges or diapers are loosely sutured across the incision, and the abdomen is secured with bandage material. The entire bandage is changed under sterile conditions every 8 hours. Primary closure is performed as drainage diminishes and the patient's condition warrants, which is usually in 3–5 days.

Complications and other considerations include:

1. While not a complication, this procedure requires rigorous nursing care. Continuous observation and sterile-bandage changes are done at least every 8 hours.
2. Hypoproteinemia. The loss of protein associated with peritonitis and open

peritoneal drainage can be significant. Intravenous supplementation of albumin and enteral or parenteral feedings may be necessary.

3. Fluid and electrolyte losses need to be carefully monitored. Twice-daily electrolyte determination, total solids/packed cell volume (TS/PCV) values, and urine output should be observed.

4. Nosocomial infections may occur easily in these patients. The challenge of providing serial sterile dressings, keeping the patient from soiling itself, and avoiding self-mutilation by the patient can be difficult. By virtue of hypoproteinemia and sepsis, these patients are immunocompromised and thus easy targets for nosocomial infection.

ILEOCECALCOLIC RESECTION AND ANASTOMOSIS

Ileocecalcolic resection and anastomosis is performed to treat intussusceptions in the ileocecal region. In addition to the postoperative concerns mentioned previously, such as infection, dehiscence, and recurrent intussusception, several others also are of concern. In association with mechanical bowel preparation and surgical bowel irritation, projectile diarrhea often may occur during anesthetic recovery or thereafter. Surgical wounds should be adequately protected and the animal kept clean. Hence, the most common postoperative complication is infection caused by contamination either from surgery or leakage. Patients are monitored closely for signs of peritonitis, with abdominocentesis performed if signs such as fever, anorexia, vomiting, abdominal pain, or distention are present.

SUBTOTAL COLECTOMY

Removal of greater than 90% of the large bowel is done to treat the feline megacolon syndrome. Loose, watery stools may be present for several weeks after a subtotal colectomy.

RECTAL PULL-THROUGH

With rectal pull-through, the distal-most rectum is incised circumferentially to allow removal, and the remaining rectum is reconstructed with perianal tissue. Surgery is performed as an aggressive means of resecting tumors or to treat severe, chronic, perianal fistulas.

Regarding postoperative care, this procedure produces pain, especially on defecation. Sidebars or an Elizabethan collar may be needed to prevent licking or biting at the rectal area.

PERIRECTAL PROCEDURES

Rectal strictures, prolapses, perianal fistulae and anal sacculitis may be treated surgically. Once again, protection from licking is very important.

Anal sac adenocarcinoma may show hypercalcemia as a paraneoplastic syndrome. Hypercalcemia is a serious medical threat that needs resolution or regulation before surgery. Signs of hypercalcemia because of malignant disease are referable to a reduction in renal function. Other tumors associated with hypercalcemia in dogs and cats include lymphoma, myeloma, mammary adenocarcinoma, tumors invading bone, and neoplasia of the parathyroid glands [14]. If during management of a postsurgical patient with one of these tumor types you become aware that preanesthesia calcium screening was not done, this should be performed in the immediate postsurgical setting to prevent renal failure and death.

ANAL SACCULECTOMY

Removal of the anal saccules is done for recurrent impaction, infection, and neoplasia. During resection, care must be taken to avoid damaging the caudal rectal nerve as well as the transverse incision in the external anal sphincter.

Postoperative concerns include:

1. Licking. Animals often lick their anal region and can produce dehiscence or infection of the anal sacculectomy incision. Judicious use of an Elizabethan collar is warranted.

2. Fecal soiling. Defecation after perianal surgery is common, and if it occurs, the perineum, if soiled, should be cleansed with soap and water and toweled dry.

3. Purse-string suture. If a suture is used to occlude temporarily the anal orifice, it must be removed after surgery. Failure to do so will produce tenesmus and dyschezia.

4. Infection. While usually not a problem in the first 24 hours after surgery, infections are common after perianal surgery. Heat, pain, swelling, or purulent incisional discharge are signs of infection.

REFERENCES

1. Spangler WL, Culbertson MK: Salivary gland disease. *J Am Vet Med Assoc* 198:465–469, 1991.
2. Leib MS, Blass CE: Gastroesophageal intussusception in the dog: a review of the literature and a case report. *JAAHA* 20:783–790, 1984.
3. Spielman BL, Shaker EH, Garvey MS: Esophageal foreign body in dogs: A retrospective study of 23 cases. *JAAHA* 28:570–574, 1992.
4. Parker NR, Walter PA, Gay J: Diagnosis and surgical management of esophageal perforation. *JAAHA* 25:587–594, 1989.
5. Ridgeway RL, Suter PF: Clinical and radiographic signs in primary and metastatic esophageal neoplasms in the dog. *J Am Vet Med Assoc* 174:700–704, 1979.
6. Whitney WD, et al: Belt loop gastropexy: technique and surgical results in 20 dogs. *JAAHA* 25:75–83, 1989.
7. Matthiesen DT: Gastric dilation volvulus syndrome. *In* Slatter D, et al, eds. Textbook of small animal surgery. Philadelphia, 1993, WB Saunders, pp. 580–593.
8. Muir WW: Gastric dilation and volvulus in the dog with emphasis on cardiac arrhythmias. *J Am Vet Med Assoc* 180:739–742, 1982.
9. O'Brien TR: Small intestine disorders in the dog and cat. Philadelphia, 1978, WB Saunders.

10. Beaumont PR: Anastomotic jejeunal ulcer secondary to gastrojejeunostomy in a dog. *JAAHA* 17:233–237, 1981.
11. Allen DA, Smeak D, Schertel EA: Prevalence of small intestine dehiscence and associated clinical factors. *JAAHA* 28:70–76, 1992.
12. Waldron DR, Hedlund CS, Pechman R: Abdominal hernias in dogs and cats. *JAAHA* 22: 817–823, 1986.
13. Boothe HW, et al: Exploratory celiotomy in 200 non-traumatized dogs and cats. *Vet Surg* 21:452–457, 1992.
14. Manten DJ: Hypercalcemia. *Vet Clin North Am* 14:891–910, 1984.

13

Surgery of the Liver and Biliary System

Hepatic surgery is performed for diagnostic procedures, to resect benign or malignant tumors, to correct portosystemic shunts, to remove calculi from the gallbladder or bile ducts, and to treat traumatic injuries to the liver and biliary tree. Surgery most often involves general anesthesia and celiotomy.

POSTSURGICAL CONCERNS OF HEPATIC SURGERY

Hepatic Function Compromise

In certain feline and canine liver diseases such as advanced cirrhosis, feline liver disease, and hepatic hypofunction because of portosystemic shunts, hepatic function can be severely compromised. The type, degree, and severity of postoperative concern in hepatobiliary surgery are directly influenced by the type of hepatobiliary disease and the procedures performed to correct or treat the problem. An otherwise healthy animal requiring a partial lobectomy following trauma may experience few postsurgical problems, whereas an animal with a portosystemic shunt or severe hepatobiliary disease can have numerous, serious postoperative problems.

Partial removal of the liver is indicated in severe trauma, neoplasia, and abscesses. The most common postoperative problem is excessive hemorrhage because of ligature failure. Animals recovering from partial hepatectomy should be monitored for signs of blood loss (see Chapter X). Hypoglycemia has been reported to occur in dogs following hepatectomy [1]. All postoperative patients either should have blood glucose levels monitored or be placed on glucose, 1 g/kg body weight/h, during surgery.

Nonregenerative anemia may be present in patients with liver disease. Decreased protein synthesis, decreased red blood cell survival, and anemia from chronic disease are possible causes.

Coagulation abnormalities also may be present. In severe, chronic hepatocellular disease, there may be insufficient hepatic production of clotting factor proteins I, II, V, VII, IX, and X. In addition, vitamin K–dependent cofactors (i.e., II, VII, IX, and X) may be depleted if biliary obstruction is present. Prothrombin and partial thromboplastin time both may be elevated. This problem should be identified presurgically.

Delayed Wound Healing

Delayed wound healing may be a problem in advanced hepatocellular disease. In cases where severe ascites is present, postoperative leakage of ascitic fluid can be troublesome and may exacerbate wound dehiscence or incisional hernia. Hypoalbuminemia may follow partial hepatectomy and result in ascites [1].

T Tubes and Percutaneous Biliary Drainage Tubes

T tubes and percutaneous biliary drainage tubes rarely are used in hepatobiliary surgery of the dog and cat. If such tubes are placed, their security and position must be maintained during recovery.

Altered Hepatic Function

With some hepatobiliary diseases, hepatic function can be compromised. Decreased clearance of anesthetics, elevations of hepatic enzyme levels, and alterations of bile acids may occur. Judicious use of drugs administered during recovery is recommended. With altered hepatic function, metabolism and conjugation of many therapeutic drugs may be altered.

Volatile Anesthetics

Certain volatile anesthetics, especially methoxyflurane, are known hepatotoxins, and their use is discouraged [2].

Infection

The hepatobiliary tree often is colonized with bacteria. *Clostridium* sp. may be present in the canine liver. Prophylactic antibiotics are recommended before surgery. Treatment of existing hepatobiliary infection is warranted should clinical signs be present or evidence of infection be observed at the time of surgery.

PANCREAS

Surgery of the pancreas is done for biopsy purposes, to remove benign or malignant tumors, and to drain pancreatic cysts and abscesses (Fig. 13–1). Considerations during postoperative care include:

1. Functional tumors of the pancreas. These may produce excessive insulin or glucagon. In these cases, it is important to monitor carefully the blood glucose levels during recovery. Insulinomas are malignant tumors with which approximately 45% of patients have regional lymphatic metastasis at the time of surgery [3]. Surgical cures for insulinoma usually are not successful.
2. Hypoglycemia. This is a common pre- and postsurgical problem. The patient is maintained on 5% dextrose solution and blood glucose levels are monitored during recovery. If complete tumor removal is achieved, euglycemia should return, and intravenous glucose administration can be stopped.
3. Intravenously administered dyes. Intravenous methylene blue is helpful in identifying insulinomas in the pancreas, and Heinz body anemia may occur if the dosage

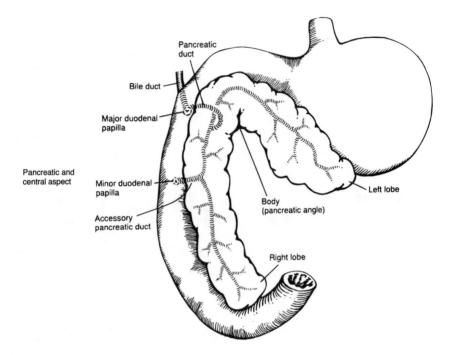

Fig. 13–1. Canine pancreatic and biliary ducts. (From Slatter D.E.: Textbook of Small Animal Surgery. Philadelphia, WB Saunders, 1985.)

is exceeded. Dyes have no systemic effect, but a blue or yellow tint to mucous membranes in the postoperative recovery place can be disconcerting [4].

4. Diabetes mellitus. This may occur as a sequela to insulinoma, pancreatic resection, or be a coexisting problem. Some general guidelines are provided for the postoperative care of diabetic patients in Table 13–1. Two important guidelines are:

A) Determine the type of insulin used and normal feeding schedule, and
B) Whenever possible, adjust the timing of surgery to fit insulin administration and feeding intervals.

Table 13–1
Guidelines for Surgery of the Patient with Diabetes Mellitus

Good control of diabetes for at least 2 to 3 weeks
Give 50% of the normal morning insulin dose 1 hour before induction
Administer a 5% dextrose solution intravenously during the procedure
Monitor blood glucose levels every 30 minutes during the procedure
Adjust fluid rate to avoid hypoglycemia
Monitor blood glucose level every 6 hours postoperatively
Give regular insulin as needed to maintain levels between 150 and 250 mg/dL
Return to normal insulin once patient is eating and drinking

(Courtesy of Douglas R. Santen, DVM)

SURGERY OF THE SPLEEN

Splenic surgery is done to repair and/or remove the traumatically injured spleen, to correct splenic torsion, and to diagnose and treat splenic tumors. In addition, splenectomy may be indicated in cases of immune-mediated hemolytic anemia or thrombocytopenia.

The spleen of the dog and cat act as a reservoir for red blood cells, with 10% or more found in the spleen [5]. The splenic reservoir helps to protect against acute blood loss as with adrenergic stimulation, where the red pulp contracts and infuses red blood cells into the systemic circulation.

In a large diagnostic survey of splenic disease [6], splenic hematoma and hyperplastic nodules were the most common reason for splenomegaly.

Splenic Hemangiosarcoma

Splenic hemangiosarcoma is the most common splenic neoplasia. Following splenectomy, dogs with this neoplasia have a median survival time of 13 weeks [7]. Unfortunately, splenectomy has little influence on survival time in animals with hemangiosarcoma. Splenectomy largely is a palliative procedure in this case.

Postoperative Care

Patients should be monitored during recovery for evidence of abdominal hemorrhage. Technical failure associated with ligature or stapling devices may result in excessive bleeding (see Chapter X). If postoperative bleeding is severe, whole-blood transfusion or reoperation may be indicated.

Dogs with splenic masses have an increased incidence of arrhythmias either pre- or postoperatively. Ventricular arrhythmias are reported to occur in 39% of dogs with hemangiosarcoma, 34% of dogs with hematoma, and 27% of dogs with leiomyosarcoma [8]. Ventricular tachycardia and premature ventricular contractions are the most common arrhythmias.

REFERENCES

1. Bjorling DE, et al: Partial hepatectomy in dogs. *Compend Cont Ed Pract Vet* 7:257–264, 1985.
2. Curtis MB: Anesthesia for gastrointestinal surgery. *In* Slatter D, ed. Textbook of small animal surgery. Philadelphia, 1993, WB Saunders, pp. 2284–2289.
3. Klauser JS, Hardy RW: Alimentary tract, liver and pancreas. *In* Slatter D, ed. Textbook of small animal surgery. Philadelphia, 1993, WB Saunders, pp. 2088–2105.
4. Orsher RJ, Rosin E: Intravenously administered dyes. *In* Slatter D, ed. Textbook of small animal surgery. Philadelphia, 1993, WB Saunders, pp. 593–612.
5. Song SH, Groom AC: The distribution of blood cells in the spleen. *Canine J Physiol Pharmacol* 49:734, 1971.
6. Johnson KA, et al: Splenomegaly in dogs. *Vet Surg* 3:160–166, 1989.
7. Spangler WL, Culbertson MR: Prevalence, type, and importance of splenic disease in dogs, 1480 cases, 1985–1989. *J Am Vet Med Assoc* 200:829–834, 1992.
8. Knapp DW, Aronsohn MG, Harpster NK: Cardiac arrhythmias associated with mass lesions of the canine spleen. *JAAHA* 29:122–128, 1993.

14

Orthopedic Procedures

CONNECTIVE TISSUES (MUSCLE, TENDONS, LIGAMENTS)

Surgical repair of muscle injuries most commonly is performed on racing breeds; however, lacerated muscles, traumatic avulsions, and other muscle injuries also occur in other breeds. In racing breeds, the gracilis muscle, long head of the triceps muscle, and tensor fascia latae are the muscles most commonly injured (Fig. 14–1), but at least 25 different muscles are reported to have sustained injuries in these animals [1].

Repair of muscle tissue requires general anesthesia with evacuation of the hematoma, careful but not overzealous debridement, and primary repair. Surgical procedures involving muscle, tendons, or ligaments produce varying levels of postoperative pain, and a pain management protocol should be developed for commonly performed procedures.

Regarding special postoperative concerns, it is important to immobilize the affected limb, if possible, for 3 weeks. The bandage and/or splint must be kept clean and dry. Also, the surgeon occasionally will use a continuous suction device to evacuate hemorrhage. If used, this device must be secured and protected from the animal.

Surgical repair of ligament or tendon injuries may involve wire, screws and washers, sutures, tissue anchors, and other orthopedic hardware. It is common to immobilize the limb postoperatively, and in many cases, an external fixateur is used to accomplish this. The fixateur must be padded to prevent lacerations, to prevent it from getting caught in the bedding, and so on.

Ligamentous injuries invariably produce joint instability or laxity, and successful repair must eliminate this. In general, few unique postoperative concerns are associated with ligament-repair surgery. If the limb is immobilized postoperatively, the bandage or splint must be kept clean and dry.

Common Ligament Injuries and Their Repair

Injuries to the anterior cruciate ligament are the most common ligamentous injuries in both the dog and the cat. There are at least 30 reported methods for treating ACL instability [2]. In general, the procedures can be divided into intra-articular and extra-articular repairs. Common and useful intraarticular repairs include the over-the-top patellar tendon technique, while the fibular head transposition and various embrication techniques are extra-articular repairs.

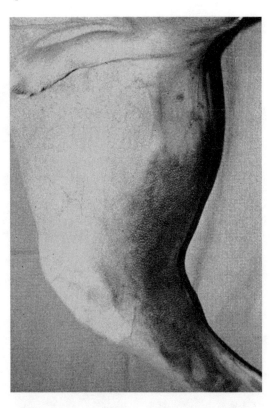

Fig. 14–1. Characteristic swelling and ecchymotic hemorrhage associated with an acute, stage-III tear of the gracilis muscle.

Specific protocols for the postoperative management of ACL repairs can be helpful, especially in practices where it is a commonly performed procedure. A suggested protocol for postoperative management of ACL would include:

1. Effective pain management, ideally beginning in the operating room near completion of the procedure.
2. Use of ice packs or a cold water–circulating blanket to reduce postsurgical swelling, inflammation, and pain (Fig. 14–2).
3. Appropriate management of bandages or splints.
4. Early use of physical therapy, including passive range of motion of the hip, stifle, and hock beginning the day after surgery.

Compartmental Syndrome

Muscle injury in a confined fascial compartment may swell because of edema, hemorrhage, or inflammation. This may result in interstitial tissue pressures that produce compression of the venous end of capillary beds, resulting in necrosis. As the pressure increases, vascular compression occurs, with ischemic necrosis of muscle as the end result. This can be an insidious process, with irreversible damage done to muscle and nerve after 4 hours of severe compression [3].

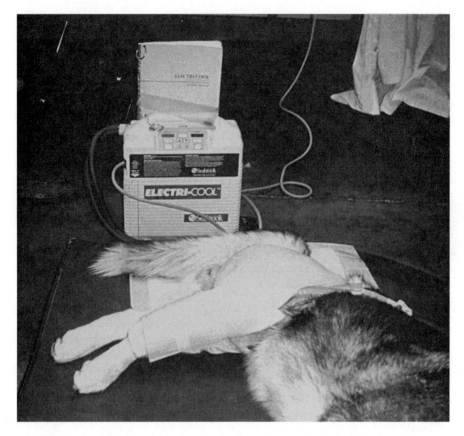

Fig. 14–2. A cold water–circulating blanket is used postoperatively following reconstruction of the anterior cruciate ligament.

Closed extremity fractures, crush wounds, and snake bites are potential causes of compartmental syndrome in the dog. Electrical injuries, thermal injuries, inappropriate use of a tourniquet, coagulopathies, overly constrictive bandages or casts, and clostridial gangrene are additional potential causes.

Compartments are areas where muscle, nerve, and blood vessels are confined within inelastic boundaries of skin, fascia, or bone. In man, at least 16 compartments are recognized, while four have been described in the dog [4–6].

The craniolateral compartment of the crus, caudal compartment of the antebrachium, caudal compartment of the crus, and the femoral compartment have been described in the dog. Normal compartmental pressures range from − 2 to 8 mm Hg, with significant necrosis of the muscle occurring at pressures over 30 mm Hg if present for over 8 hours. Clinical signs of compartmental syndrome include a swollen, painful leg with tense, painful muscle. Diminished distal-nerve function and pulse compromise also may be present. Compartmental pressures can be monitored with a Stryker Wick Catheter [Stryker Co., Kalamazoo, MI.] (Fig. 14–3). A tentative diagnosis based on clinical signs or increased compartmental pressure may warrant a compartmental fasciotomy.

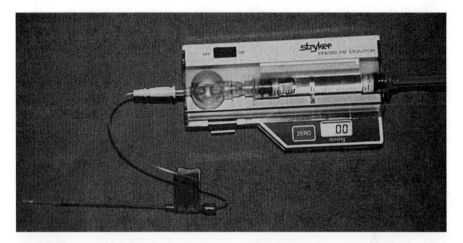

Fig. 14–3. A commercially available Wick catheter for measuring and monitoring compartmental pressure. (Stryker Intracompartmental Pressure Monitor, Stryker Surgical, Kalamazoo, Mich.)

FRACTURE REPAIR

Surgical repair of fractures is a common procedure in many practices. As with most commonly performed procedures, an established protocol for postsurgical care can be developed by the surgical staff to ensure solid, standardized care. Such a protocol should include pain management, supervised recovery from anesthesia, initial physical therapy, attention to the physical needs of the patient (i.e., need for water, facilitation of urination and defecation, food), and management of protective bandages or splints.

A suggested postoperative femoral fracture protocol would be:

1. Pain control begins in the operating room at the time of skin closure. Butorphanol, 0.8–1.2 mg/kg body weight, or ketolorac, 0.15 mg/kg, are suggested.
2. Pull the intravenous catheter when the patient is fully conscious, and discontinue fluids.
3. Apply ice packs to the surgical extremity during recovery from anesthesia.
4. Begin passive range of motion exercises as patient tolerance allows.
5. Keep the incisional area clean and dry.
6. Provide assistance when necessary to help the animal urinate and defecate.

SURGICAL PROCEDURES OF THE FORELIMB

Orthopedic procedures of the forelimb are common and range from routine fracture repair to sophisticated limb salvage for cancer treatment. The forelimbs of domestic quadripeds bear 60% of their body weight, and coupled with the problems inherent in immobilization of postoperative scapular or humeral fractures, this creates challenges for early mobility and immobilization.

It is important to protect the wound for at least 48 hours to minimize bacterial contamination [7]. Compartmental syndrome is less common in the postoperative setting, but an index of suspicion during recovery is helpful. Biting or licking the cast or bandage is not helpful and may be a sign of discomfort resulting from a poorly placed or overly tight bandage or cast. In general, when a patient persists in biting or licking a cast or bandage, it should be taken as a sign that a problem exists. To address it, one should remove the bandage, splint, or cast, and examine the surgical site as well as the entire extremity. If judged to be normal, the bandage may be replaced. Judicious use of an Elizabethan collar or immobilizing bandage may be used at this juncture.

Casting of forelimb fractures is a means of providing primary or secondary immobilization. A tenet of internal fixation of fractures is that the fracture repair is stable enough to "stand alone," minimizing the need for cast immobilization. In spite of this, casts often are added as a secondary means of stability. Casting of the forelimb is done for orthopedic injuries distal to the elbow and rarely is effective for scapular or humeral fractures. Some important concerns regarding castings include:

1. Use two to four layers of cast padding, distributed evenly over the limb, and avoid roll cotton. Give particular attention to the areas of the olecranon and accessory carpal bone (Fig. 14–4).

2. Apply all materials with the limb in the desired position for casting. If the limb is being casted in 45° of carpal flexion, all layers of padding should be applied with the limb held in this location (Fig. 14–5).

3. Do not leave distal aspects of the extremity uncasted, because edema quickly forms. It is advisable to leave a distal opening through which to inspect the toes.

4. When possible, protect the distal end of the cast with a walking bar (Fig. 14–6) to prevent soiling and destruction of the cast.

5. Consider applying the cast while the animal is still recovering from general anesthesia. A completely relaxed patient greatly facilitates this procedure.

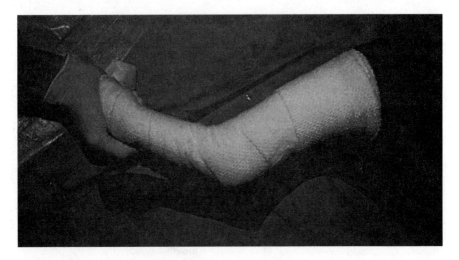

Fig. 14–4. Two to four layers of padding are applied before casting to protect the leg. (Courtesy of David M. Ennis, DVM.)

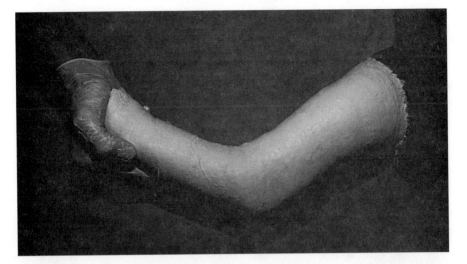

Fig. 14–5. The cast padding and material are applied with the limb in the desired position. This minimizes wrinkles or areas of incisional pressure that may lead to skin or tissue necrosis. (Courtesy of David M. Ennis, DVM.)

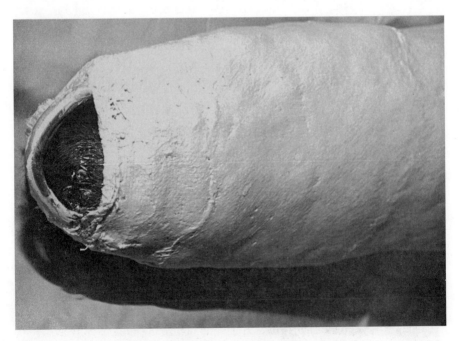

Fig. 14–6. The cast padding and material cover the entire extremity, with a small hole distally for visualization and palpation of the toes. An aluminum walking bar has been incorporated into this cast. (Courtesy of David M. Ennis, DVM.)

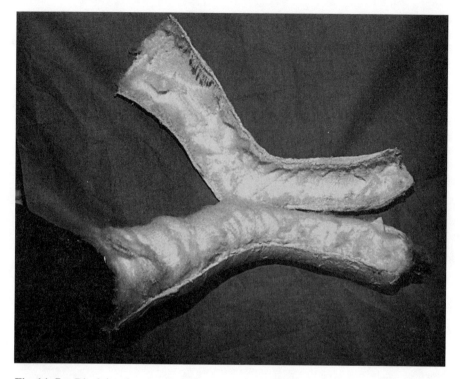

Fig. 14–7. Bivalving the cast allows for easy removal and inspection should swelling occur. (Courtesy of David M. Ennis, DVM.)

6. Consider bivalving the cast for the first 24 to 48 hours (Fig. 14–7) so that it can be removed easily should excessive swelling or discomfort occur.

7. When in doubt about a cast's excessive tightness, the animal persistently chews at it, or it becomes soiled, remove the cast immediately to allow inspection of the extremity and recasting.

8. A carefully applied cast should provide postoperative support and comfort to the patient. In most cases, casts are well tolerated.

9. In summary, be aware of signs from the patient indicating discomfort or an improperly applied cast. An index of suspicion coupled with a willingness to remove and subsequently replace a cast is mandatory. Biting or chewing, persistent panting or fever, odiferous discharge, or excessive swelling of the toes indicate potential trouble. Failure to recognize casting problems may result in loss of soft tissues and greatly exacerbate normal healing. In severe cases, loss of the limb may result.

ORTHOPEDIC PROCEDURES OF THE PELVIS

Pelvic surgery is performed to reduce and immobilize fractures, to correct osseous malunion, to reform the coxofemoral joint, and to collect bone marrow for analysis. The soft-tissue structures within the pelvic canal include the bladder, urethra, colon, pelvic blood vessels, and nerves, and these structures are prone to injury because of existing trauma or surgery. From 20% to 30% [8] of all fractures in the dog involve the pelvis, and as many as 60% have other associated injuries. Of these injuries, 56% involve the musculoskeletal system, 23% the abdomen and thorax, and 20% the nervous system [9] (Table 14–1).

Areas of concern following pelvic surgery include:

1. Thoracic injuries. Common thoracic injuries following pelvic trauma are pulmonary contusion, pneumothorax, and pleural effusion. As many as 50% of dogs and 15% of cats with pelvic injury also have thoracic injuries [8]. Survey radiographs of the thorax and abdomen should be standard procedure with pelvic injury.

2. Peripheral nerve damage. Close proximity of the lumbosacral plexus, femoral, sciatic, and pudendal nerves make them uniquely susceptible to bone fragments or

Table 14–1
Soft-Tissue Conditions Associated with Pelvic Fractures

Abdominal injuries
  Abdominal hernia
  Avulsion of the bladder neck from the urethra
  Avulsion of the ureter
  Bladder herniation
  Bladder mucosa damage
  Bladder rupture
  Bowel necrosis
  Bowel perforation
  Mesenteric damage and ischemia
  Rectal tear
  Ruptured gallbladder and common bile duct
  Ruptured parenchymatous organs
  Urethral rupture

Cardiovascular conditions
  Iliac arterial hemorrhage
  Myocardial ischemia and contusion

Peripheral nerve damage
  Avulsion of lumbosacral roots
  Femoral nerve injury
  Lumbosacral trunk injury
  Sacral roots and pelvic plexus injury
  Sciatic nerve injury

Thoracic injuries
  Diaphragmatic hernia
  Pleural effusion and/or hemothorax
  Pneumothorax
  Pulmonary contusion

Other soft-tissue injuries
  Contusion
  Hemorrhage
  Laceration

(From Verslraete, FJM: Dx. of Soft Tissue Injuries Associated with Pelvic Fractures. Comp. Cont. Ed., (14)7;1992.)

iatrogenic injury from bone clamps, screws, and other hardware. These may produce nerve avulsion or direct damage to the nerve itself. Nerve function should be assessed before surgery to provide a comparison for postoperative recovery. Significant changes in nerve function and motor or sensory abilities are reasons for great concern. Sciatic-nerve entrapment may occur as a delayed sequela to pelvic fractures.

3. Hemorrhage from pelvic fractures or surgery. This can be substantial and may become life-threatening with preexisting coagulopathies. When in doubt, serial total solids and packed cell volume can be done. Fluid replacement, colloids, or packed red blood cells may be needed (see Chapter X).

4. Bowel and bladder function. With severe pelvic canal injuries, the bowel, bladder, and lower urinary tract are jeopardized. Sharp bone fragments may lacerate these structures at the time of injury, and the full extent of damage may not be readily apparent. Before surgery, a rectal exam should be performed and the animal's ability to urinate determined. Rectal perforation is rare (four cases reported out of 600 pelvic fractures) but is a devastating injury, especially if it is initially undetected [10]. In many instances, a contrast cystogram and urethrogram are needed to rule out or verify injuries. Urinary trauma may include bladder laceration or rupture, urethral laceration, ureter avulsion, and renal trauma. In severe pelvic trauma, the bladder may herniate caudally, into the pelvic canal, through a tear in the rectal wall, a tear in the abdominal wall, or the prostatic symphisis. With some urethral lacerations, it is possible for the animal to form a urinary stream but still sustain periurethral leakage.

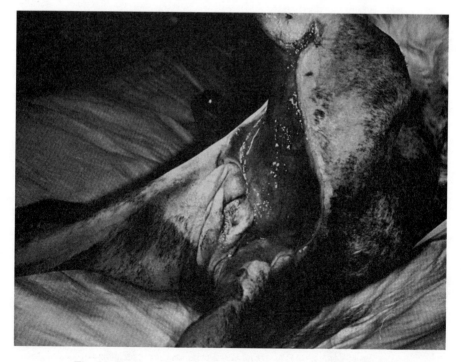

Fig. 14–8.   Extensive skin loss following massive pelvic trauma.

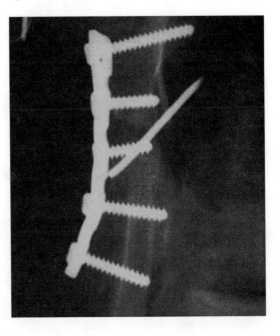

Fig. 14–9. This Steinman pin is too long and may intrude into the pelvic canal.

5. Skin loss and tissue necrosis. Significant vascular damage and tissue trauma may be present in some pelvic injuries. The full extent of injury may be apparent only after several days (Fig. 14–8).

6. Licking. Dogs and cats have unlimited access to incisions made about the pelvis. This may be more problematic with multiple wounds. An Elizabethan collar or use of a noxious deterrent may be needed.

7. Placement of pins, wires, and screws. When orthopedic hardware is used to reconstruct the pelvis, its exact location and size must be determined. It is possible to place screws or pins inadvertently through the sacroiliac joint into the spinal canal, or have screws that are too long impinge on pelvic canal structures (Fig. 14–9). The mandatory need for two postoperative radiographic views of any reconstructive surgery is obvious.

ORTHOPEDIC PROCEDURES OF THE HINDLIMB

The spectrum of procedures involving the hindlimb varies from simple phalangeal luxations to total joint replacement. General areas of concern are pain management, protection of the surgical wound, and attention to blood loss (see Chapters IV, VI and X).

Nerve Damage

Iatrogenic injuries of the sciatic nerve have been described with both open and closed pinning of femoral fractures. Sciatic-nerve injury can occur with femoral-head excision, pin placement in proximal and distal femoral fractures, and from callous impingement following fracture healing (Fig. 14–10). This may be obvious

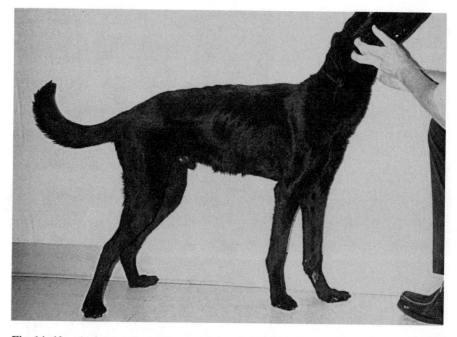

Fig. 14–10. An iatrogenic, sciatic-nerve injury following intramedullary pinning of a femoral fracture. (Courtesy of Steven B. Colter, DVM.)

immediately after surgery, with the animal showing extraordinary pain near the proximal femur. Anterior ventral coxofemoral luxations may injure the femoral nerve, and procedures cranial to the acetabulum may produce iatrogenic femoral-nerve injuries. Fibular head transposition done for ACL repair may produce peroneal nerve injuries.

Compartmental Syndrome

The femoral compartment is susceptible to injury in traumatic femoral fractures. It is a rare phenomenon postsurgically, but compartmental syndrome and attendant damage may be present before surgery. Quadriceps tiedown seen after distal femoral fractures may be in part a compartmental injury.

Physical Therapy

A physical therapy protocol may begin in the hours after surgery. Such a protocol might include ice packs or other means of cooling along the incision site, passive range of motion, and gentle massage or rotation.

Ambulation

Animals with orthopedic injuries or procedures of one hindlimb are faster to ambulate than those with forelimb problems. Of special concern are those patients with several injured limbs or pelvic fractures. These patients are at risk for decubital

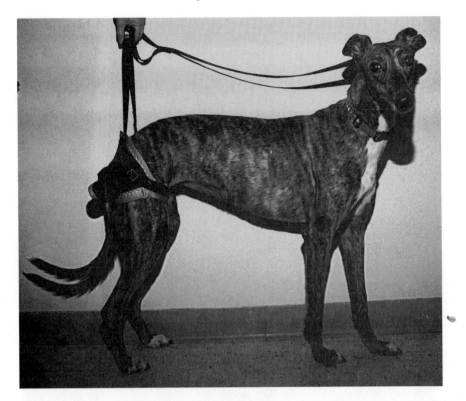

Fig. 14–11.   This sling (Walkabout™, Santa Cruz, CA. Walkabout Harnesses Co. Designer: *Cathy Erwin*.) can be useful in helping early ambulation. (Courtesy of David M. Ennis, DVM.)

ulcers, urine scalding, and fecal soilage. Use of cage grates, a water bed, fleece blanket, or other measures may be needed during recovery and convalescence. These patients also may need assistance in ambulating with a sling device (Fig. 14–11).

PELVIC SURGERY

Corrective procedures for canine hip dysplasia are commonly performed. These range from corrective osteotomies in young animals with dysplastic conformation to total hip replacement in dogs with coxofemoral degenerative joint disease.

Corrective osteotomy:

Pelvic osteotomy to allow rotation of the acetabular segment and subtrochanteric osteotomy of the femur are performed in young dogs with dysplastic conformation. Triple pelvic osteotomy currently is the most commonly performed. This procedure involves osteotomy of the pubis, ischium, and ilium through three separate incisions. Following the osteotomies, the isolated acetabular segment is rotated. Specially designed plates (Slocum Plates, Slocum Industries, Eugene, OR) that allow for 20°, 30°, or 45° of correction are available (Fig. 14–12). Alternatively available are

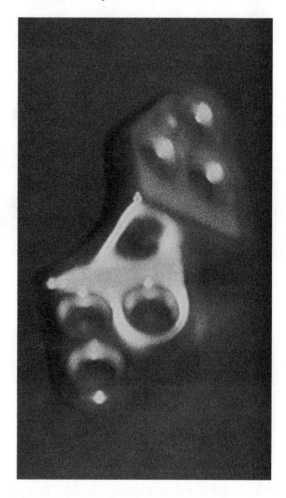

Fig. 14–12. A prebended bone plate has rotated the acetabular segment by 30°.

bone plates such as the 3.5-mm dynamic compression plate (DCP) or 4.5-mm DCP (Synthes, Paoli, PA), which may be bent by hand to a desired angle of correction.

Triple pelvic osteotomy can be technically challenging and carries some risk for surgical iatrogenesis. Postoperative complications do occur, and these include:

1. Hemorrhage. In the hemostatically healthy patient, severe hemorrhage is rare. We have encountered several patients with persistent hemorrhage from incised nutrient foramina on the ischium. This hemorrhage resulted in a large hematoma and required reoperation to stop the bleeding. It is possible to damage the cranial gluteal artery when approaching the iliac wing, and there is a large nutrient vessel associated with the cranial ventral aspect of the iliac wing.

2. Nerve damage. Damage to the obturator, femoral, and sciatic nerves may occur with triple pelvic osteotomy. Once anesthetic recovery has occurred, nerve-specific

reflexes should be checked to ensure their integrity. In a study of twenty triple pelvic osteotomies, neurologic deficits constituted 3% of complications [11].

3. Self-mutilation. Multiple osteotomies are painful, and with poor pain-management procedures, licking and self-mutilation are common. For some reason, the ischiatic incision is most commonly involved. Judicious pain management and Elizabethan-collar application are advisable.

4. Pelvic canal compromise. When the triple pelvic osteotomy is done bilaterally, it is possible to greatly reduce the circumference of the pelvic canal. In addition, medial rotation of both pubic bones may compromise the pelvic urethra. These problems may not be evident in the first 24 hours following surgery, and the animal should be observed urinating or defecating before discharge. A rectal examination should be performed postoperatively as well.

5. Bone plate disruption. When excessive early ambulation occurs, the bone screws that secure the plate may fail, allowing the plate to move away from the cranial or caudal segment (Fig. 14–13). When this occurs in the immediate postoperative period, it requires immediate reoperation. Implant loosening can be a frequent occurrence following triple pelvic osteotomy, with rates as high as 50% [11].

6. Other reported problems following triple pelvic osteotomy are incisional problems, acetabular fracture, iliopsoas pain, urethral impingement, and inadequate reduction of ilial osteotomies.

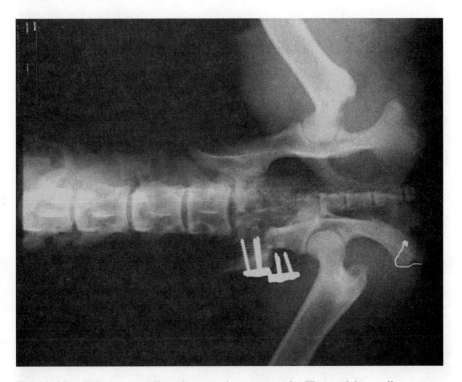

Fig. 14–13. This dog was allowed to exercise prematurely. The caudal cancellous screws lost their purchase, allowing the osteotomy to disrupt.

The suggested postoperative protocol for triple pelvic osteotomy is:

1. Place ice packs on the incisions during recovery. Then apply ice packs four times daily during hospitalization.
2. The operated leg should be cycled through its normal passive range of motion beginning the day of surgery and then three times daily for the first week following surgery.
3. Assisted walking with towels or Walkabout [Walkabout Harnesses Co., Santa Cruz, CA, Designer: Cathy Erwin] as needed.
4. Appropriate pain management (see Chapter VI).

Total Hip Replacement

Total hip replacement involves osteotomy of the femoral head and neck and the placement of a prosthesis into the femoral canal. The prosthesis may be cemented with methylmethacrylate, or it may be fitted into the femur without cement. Almost all clinical cases of total hip replacement in the dog use cemented prostheses. The cartilage and subchondral bone in the acetabulum are removed with bone reamers, and the polypropylene acetabulum is cemented in the bone.

Possible complications of this procedure include:

1. Hemorrhage. A craniolateral approach to the coxofemoral joint is used for total hip replacement; excessive hemorrhage is unusual. Many total hip recipients are older and should be screened presurgically for preexisting metabolic disease.

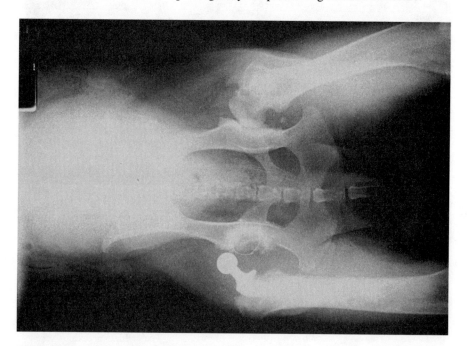

Fig. 14–14. Postoperative coxofemoral luxation that occurred when the dog slipped on a slick floor and both legs were severely abducted.

2. Nerve damage. Excessive traction may traumatize the sciatic nerve. Nerve damage has been reported in 5 of 22 cases [12] and may range from mild neuropraxia to complete nerve transection.

3. Luxation. It is possible to luxate the hip following total hip replacement. This may occur postoperatively if the patient walks on a slick floor and the leg is severely abducted (Fig. 14–14). Assisted walking with a towel or Walkabout is recommended following surgery. Persistent or recurrent luxation usually indicates a technical error in the position of the prosthesis, most often the acetabular component. Reoperation and replacement of the prosthesis often is required.

4. Infection. While rare, this is a devastating complication with cemented total hip replacement. It is imperative that self-mutilation be prohibited and scrupulous wound care provided after surgery to prevent wound infection.

The suggested postoperative protocol for total hip replacement is:

1. Ice packs are applied during anesthetic recovery and then four times daily thereafter.
2. The operated leg should be cycled through its normal passive range of motion following surgery and continued three times daily for the first week following surgery.
3. Assisted postoperative walking with towels or a Walkabout.

REFERENCES

1. Taylor RA: Muscle and tendon injuries of canine athletes. *In* Proceedings 1992 ACVS Veterinary Symposium. Miami, 1992, ACVS Veterinary Symposium, pp. 549–551. *Publ Amer Coll Vet Surgeons.*
2. Taylor RA: Selected table topics: arthroscopy and partial cruciate tears, Sept. 9, 1992, 9870 E. Alameda Ave., Denver, CO. 80209.
3. Ross D: Acute compartmental syndrome. *Orthop Nurs* 10:33, 1991.
4. de Haan JJ, Beale BS: Compartment syndrome in the dog. *JAAHA* 29:134–140, 1993.
5. Basinger RR, et al: Osteofascial compartment syndrome in the dog. *Vet Surg* 16:427–434, 1987.
6. Olivieri M, Suter P: Compartmental syndrome of the front leg of a dog due to rupture of the median artery. *JAAHA* 14:210–218, 1978.
7. Coit DG, Sclafani L: Care of the surgical wound. *In* Wilmore DW, et al, editors. Care of the Surgical Patient. *Sci Am Med* 2:1–10.
8. Verstraete FJM, Lambrechts NE: Diagnosis of soft tissue injury associated with pelvic fractures. *Compend Cont Ed Pract Vet* 14:921–931, 1992.
9. Brasmer TH: The Acutely Traumatized Small Animal Patient. Philadelphia, 1984, WB Saunders.
10. Lewis DD, et al: Rectal perforations associated with pelvic fractures and sacroiliac fracture separations in 4 dogs. *JAAHA* 28:175–181, 1992.
11. Remedios AM, Fries CL: Implant complications in 20 triple pelvic osteotomies, veterinary and comparative orthopaedics and traumatology. 1993, FK Schattauer, pp. 27–32.
12. Olmstead ML, Hohn BR, Turner TM: A five year study of 221 total hip replacements in the dog. *JAVMA* 183:191–194, 1983.

15

Surgery of the Genitourinary System

Organs of the genitourinary system are frequent targets of operation. Surgical procedures may be done for diagnostic purposes, to evaluate and treat traumatic injury, to remove calculi, or to remove an organ such as the kidney or uterus. Anesthetic agents may have a profound effect on renal function. If anesthetic-induced hypotension occurs, some degree of renal vasoconstriction also may occur. Anesthetic agents containing fluoride metabolites can produce nephrotoxicity. Methoxyfluorane, given alone or in combination with postoperative nonsteroidal anti-inflammatory drug (NSAID) analgesia, can result in high-output renal failure [1]. Acute renal failure caused by contrast media (diatrizoate meglumine and diatrizoate sodium) following a presurgical evaluation that included an intravenous pyelogram (IVP) has been reported [2].

KIDNEYS

Trauma

Pelvic trauma frequently occurs in small animals. The retroperitoneal location of the kidneys affords some protection; however, because of its looser suspension, the left kidney is more susceptible to contusion and laceration. Patients with severe renal trauma have associated abdominal and skeletal injuries. In cases of renal trauma, an in-depth, presurgical examination can help to predict the outcome and extent of injury. Tests may include urinalysis, renal biochemical profile (sodium, potassium, blood urea nitrogen, creatinine), plain and contrast radiography, and ultrasound.

Renal trauma has been classified into four groups:

Class I: subcapsular hematoma,
Class II: capsular tear,
Class III: renal trauma including the pelvis, and,
Class IV: massive hilar–parenchyma damage.

Often, class III and IV injuries require unilateral nephrectomy.

In terms of special postoperative concerns, these patients should be monitored and evaluated for blood loss and maintenance of normal blood pressure. Preservation of renal function is important, so a closed urinary catheter often is maintained to measure both urinary output and volume. Aggressive support of the patient's fluid and electrolyte needs is important. Developing a flow chart to chronicle fluid administration and urine production (ins/outs) can be helpful. These patients also may have abdominal drains placed to drain hematomas or to prevent seromas from forming.

In general, certain antibiotic agents may be nephrotoxic, and of particular concern are the aminoglycosides. Potentially nephrotoxic antibiotics are:

Amikacin,
Gentamicin,
Tobramycin,
Tetracycline (associated with degradation products from outdated tetracycline),
Streptomycin,
Kanamycin,
Polymyxin, and
Cephaloridine.

Certain NSAIDs may be nephrotoxic as well. Of particular concern is acetaminophen in cats and flunixin meglumine in combination with methoxyfluorane in dogs.

Nephrectomy

Nephrectomy may be indicated for extensive trauma, renal abscesses, renal or perirenal cysts, ureteral ectopia, unilateral hydronephrosis, renal parasites, neoplasia, and severe pyelonephritis. Special postoperative concerns involve careful monitoring for renal function and blood loss. If an associated contralateral renal, ureteral, bladder, or urethral repair existed, one should be aware of possible leakage of urine. Periodic determination of serum electrolytes, urinalysis, and blood urea nitrogen/creatinine values should be performed. Serial determination of packed cell volume, total solids, and blood pressure measurement are advisable when uncontrolled hemorrhage may be present.

Elective nephrectomy is classified as a clean–contaminated procedure, and prophylactic antibiotics are indicated. Ideally, a suitable broad-spectrum drug is bolused just before surgery so that bacteriocidal levels of the antibiotic are present in the tissues during the procedure. In cases with known or suspected infection or those with massive trauma, treatment with appropriate antibiotics should be started before surgery and continue for a minimum of 7 to 10 days.

Nephrotomy

Nephrotomy usually is performed for the removal of renal calculi. Medical treatment of renal calculi often is unsuccessful, and it is not possible to eliminate a urinary tract infection without removing the renal calculi. This is not a benign procedure, as there may be a temporary decrease of 20% to 50% in renal function [3]. Maximum impairment of renal function can occur 3 weeks after surgery. Furthermore, 33% of nephrotomy cases in the study by Gahring et al [3] had postoperative complications such as pyelonephritis or recurrence of renal calculi.

Careful presurgical assessment of renal function, hydration status and if possible, identification of urinary tract pathogens should be done. Appropriate antimicrobial therapy, correction of uremia, electrolyte imbalances, and acid–base status are important considerations. Continuous hydration and diuresis must be maintained during and after the procedure.

Plain and contrast radiography are helpful presurgical evaluations. An IVP should be done to evaluate renal function, especially in cases of bilateral nephroliths or radiolucent nephroliths. It is possible to have a unilateral nephrolith, a radiographically normal contralateral kidney, normal renal function tests, and the IVP to show that the only functioning kidney is the one with the nephrolith. Failure to evaluate adequately both kidneys before surgery can lead to disaster. Ultrasonic imaging is a useful alternative to conventional radiography and is equally effective.

In some cases, pyelolithotomy may be performed instead of nephrotomy [4]. While more technically demanding, this procedure results in less renal parynchemal damage. Nephrotomy closure may be done with multiple capsular sutures, or the two halves of the kidney may be manually compressed for 5 minutes to allow fibrin adhesion to hold the tissue together.

Postoperative Concerns

Persistent hematuria may continue for several days following nephrotomy. To promote diuresis, intravenous fluids may flush out clotting factors in the urine.

In the hemostatically healthy patient, extensive hemorrhage following conventional or sutureless nephrotomy is not a problem. The coagulated blood from the incision helps to glue the two renal halves together.

Renal Biopsy

This is a commonly performed diagnostic procedure. Samples may be taken with trucut needles or by surgical excision of renal tissue. Often, this is done on patients with existing renal pathology using chemical restraint and local anesthesia. Renal biopsy can be accomplished with standard laparoscopic methods, and this technique allows directed visualization of the biopsy site. We have observed severe postrenal biopsy hemorrhage that necessitated a nephrectomy to control the hemorrhage.

Ultrasound-guided needle biopsy is a safe procedure. In 70 cases, there were five minor complications, such as immediate localized hemorrhage, and one with major perirenal hemorrhage causing the packed cell volume to drop to 20% [5].

Special Concerns

As with other renal surgical procedures, concern about blood loss and maintenance of renal function exists. Diuresis, periodic assessment of urine production, blood pressure, packed cell volume, and total solids should be done. In animals with known or suspected coagulopathies, a presurgical coagulation profile, platelet count, and assay of factor VIII R:Ag can be helpful, as can a buccal mucosal bleeding time.

UROGENITAL SURGERY

Surgery of the lower urogenital system is done to alleviate urinary obstruction at the ureter, bladder, or urethral level. In addition, correction of anatomic defects such as ectopic ureters and uterus masculinis may be done surgically. Tumor biopsy and removal as well as a host of procedures for both male and female genitalia and sex organs also are commonly performed.

URETERS

The ureters may be lacerated by trauma or avulsed from the bladder. They may be obstructed with calculi or tumor or be lacerated iatrogenically by an inexperienced surgeon. In some animals, the ureters enter the bladder in an ectopic location, such as the bladder neck or urethra, and produce urinary incontinence. Ectopic ureters are more frequent in female dogs. Transitional cell carcinoma of the bladder may extend to include the ureters.

Problems unique to ureteral surgery include:

1. Removal or dislodgement of ureteral catheters placed postsurgically to stent and drain the ureters. Some surgeons prefer to place ureteral catheters during surgery, and they should be well secured externally and connected to a sterile urine-collection system.

2. Iatrogenic injuries such as lacerations or ligation may not be apparent immediately after surgery. With laceration, some degree of uroperitoneal fluid develops, with associated electrolyte and acid–base abnormalities. With ligation, this problem may be apparent only through specialized tests such as ultrasound or an excretory urogram.

3. Partial ureteral obstruction also may occur following repair of ureteral lacerations or reimplantation of the ureter into the bladder. This may result from mucosal edema, blood clots, or excessive tissue trauma. When this occurs at the ureterovesicular junction, some degree of hydroureter may exist.

4. Many animals with ureteral ectopia have an existing urinary tract infection [6]. In one group of ectopic-ureter animals, 64% had positive bacterial cultures from urine samples taken at the time of surgery [7]. If antibiotic therapy is begun during surgery, it should be continued postoperatively.

5. While ureteral stenosis usually is not evident in the immediate postsurgical period, this is a frequent sequela to ureteral surgery.

6. Urinary leakage most often occurs in the early postsurgical period (i.e., 1–3 days).

7. Ureteral surgery may disturb normal ureteral peristalsis, and some degree of hydroureter or hydronephrosis may occur. Without other contributing factors, this usually resolves in 2 to 6 weeks.

URINARY BLADDER

Bladder surgery is performed to remove cystic calculi, repair ruptures or lacerations, and treat ectopic ureters. Bladder surgery also is done to biopsy, evaluate, and possibly remove cysts, polyps, benign tumors, and malignant cancer (most notably transitional cell carcinoma). The bladder may be retroflexed into the hernial sac of perineal hernias, and obstruction may result.

Urinary tract trauma is often present with pelvic injuries. Of 100 dogs studied by Selcer [8], 39 had concurrent urinary tract trauma. In this group also were four unrelated avulsions and three cases of hydroureter. Because of increased intra-abdominal pressure following blunt trauma, the bladder may rupture. Sharp bone fragments may pierce the bladder or urethra, and severe bruising of the bladder wall may lead to bladder-wall necrosis. In one study [9], pelvic fractures accounted for

46% of all bladder ruptures documented. With bladder rupture, urine leakage occurs in the peritoneal cavity.

URETHRA

Urethral surgery is done to repair lacerations, remove uroliths, and resect both benign and malignant tumors. Less frequent urethral problems are urethral prolapse (which most commonly occurs in young brachiocephalic breeds), hypospadias, urethral diverticlum or fistulae, and fractures of the os penis. Pelvic-fracture fragments may lacerate the membraneous urethra, and urethral injuries also may result from gunshots, bite wounds, or iatrogenic causes.

Special postoperative concerns include:

1. Licking. In many cases, a urinary catheter is placed during or immediately after surgery. It is important that the catheter is securely placed and the patient not allowed to chew, lick at, or dislodge it. In cases of trauma or rupture, there may be subcutaneous extravasation of urine, which is very irritating and may cause excessive licking.

2. With perineal urethrostomy in the cat, use either shredded paper or crumbled styrofoam instead of earthen litter for the first several days following surgery.

3. Bladder expression. Beginning soon after surgery, it may be necessary to express the bladder gently, especially if no urethral catheter is in place (Fig. 15–1).

4. Fluid and electrolyte needs. It is crucial to monitor both fluids and electrolytes during the postoperative period.

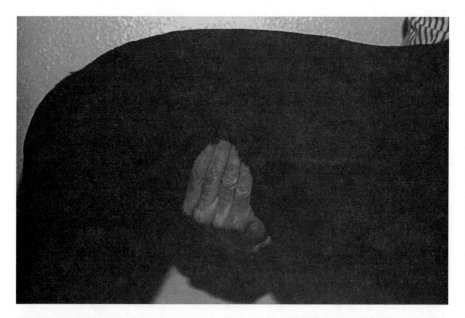

Fig. 15–1. When bladder expression is ordered, the animal is supported and the bladder gently compressed. It is helpful to apply slow, firm pressure. (Courtesy of David M. Ennis, DVM).

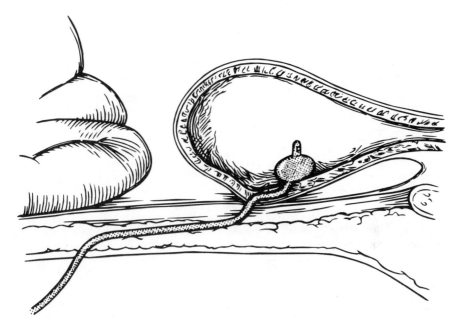

Fig. 15–2. A tube cystopexy to allow easy urinary diversion. (From JAAHA, 25(3), 1989, p. 32)

5. Urinary output. This parameter is easily measured if an indwelling catheter is present; if not, the output may be estimated.

6. Infection. Prolonged catheterization and trauma associated with the injury may predispose the site to infection. Continuation of appropriate antimicrobial therapy is recommended.

7. Closed urinary-drainage system. When prolonged catheterization or use of a urethral stent is anticipated, a sterilely placed urinary catheter, connected via sterile tubing and collection bag, is advisable. Care in the management of the system will minimize urinary infection. As an alternative, tube cytopexy (Fig. 15–2) can be used to drain urine and temporarily bypass the urethra. Great care must be taken to ensure that the tube is not dislodged, because significant uroperitoneum or extravasation of urine subcutaneously will occur. This may be an occult problem with no evidence of abdominal distention. Assessment of renal output, urinalysis, and periodic examination of serum and abdominal fluid electrolytes, urea nitrogen, and creatinine can be helpful.

8. Hematuria. Persistent hematuria can occur after surgery or trauma of the urinary tract. Table 15–1 is helpful in determining the site of urinary-tract hemorrhage.

UTERUS AND OVARIES

Ovariohysterectomy is the most commonly performed surgical procedure in many small-animal practices. All too often, however, these procedures are relegated to the youngest and most inexperienced surgeon. The procedure may be quick and easy

Table 15-1
Urinary Findings in Glomerular and Extraglomerular Bleeding

Urinary finding	Glomerular bleeding	Extraglomerular bleeding
Red-cell casts	May be present	Absent
Red-cell morphology	Dysmorphic	Uniform
Proteinuria		
>500 mg	May be present	Absent
With gross bleeding	Red or brown	Red
Clots	Absent	May be present

(With permission from Rose, BD: Approach to the Patient with Renal Disease. Section 10, III, p. 10. Scientific American Medicine, Rubenstein, E and Federman, DD, editors, New York, 1989.)

in a small, prepubescent animal, but it is exceedingly difficult in a large, deep-chested, older female.

There are other surgical diseases of the ovaries and uterus as well. These include ovarion and uterine neoplasia. Uterine torsion or rupture can occur in the gravid uterus or in cases of pyometra. Uterine prolapse also can occur in the postpartum period. In addition, cesarean section may be done as an elective or emergency procedure.

Hemorrhage

Unnoticed intraabdominal hemorrhage is the most common cause of postoperative deaths. Ligatures may slip, knots come untied, or hemorrhage occur during recovery as blood pressure returns to normal. It is necessary to observe these patients carefully for signs of hemorrhage.

Septic Shock

Many middle- to older-aged female dogs and cats develop pyometra, which is a pus-filled uterus that may or may not drain via the caudal genitourinary tract. Pyometra is a disease that occurs during the diestrus period of the estrus cycle. The most common organism cultured from the uterus is *Escherichia coli,* but many other aerobic and anaerobic organisms may be present. Pyometra is a systemic disease, and patients often present with acidosis, azotemia, leukocytosis, hyperglobulinemia, and anemia. Death rates of 5% for dogs and 8% for cats have been documented, with most deaths attributed to sepsis [10,11].

Patients recovering from an ovariohysterectomy for pyometra should be monitored carefully. Hypotension, hypoglycemia, hypothermia, and leukopenia are signs of developing sepsis. Several criteria that may indicate early septic shock are:

Tachycardia
Tachypnea
Decreased platelet count
Hypotension
Abnormal body temperature
Abnormal white-blood-cell count, and
Presence of a septic focus.

Table 15-2
Priorities in the Treatment of Septic Shock

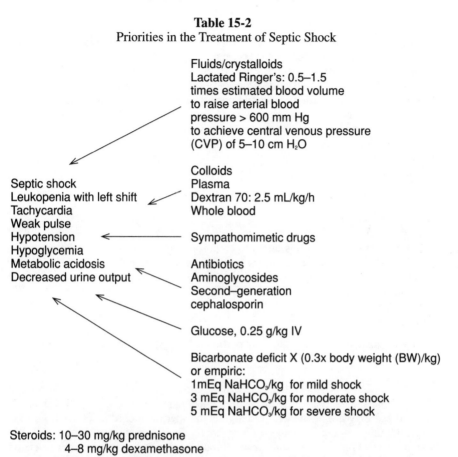

Septic shock
Leukopenia with left shift
Tachycardia
Weak pulse
Hypotension
Hypoglycemia
Metabolic acidosis
Decreased urine output

Fluids/crystalloids
Lactated Ringer's: 0.5–1.5
times estimated blood volume
to raise arterial blood
pressure > 600 mm Hg
to achieve central venous pressure
(CVP) of 5–10 cm H_2O

Colloids
Plasma
Dextran 70: 2.5 mL/kg/h
Whole blood

Sympathomimetic drugs

Antibiotics
Aminoglycosides
Second–generation
cephalosporin

Glucose, 0.25 g/kg IV

Bicarbonate deficit X (0.3x body weight (BW)/kg)
or empiric:
1mEq $NaHCO_3$/kg for mild shock
3 mEq $NaHCO_3$/kg for moderate shock
5 mEq $NaHCO_3$/kg for severe shock

Steroids: 10–30 mg/kg prednisone
4–8 mg/kg dexamethasone

(From Haskins, S.C.: Management of Septic Shock: Symposia. JAVMA, 1992;
(200) 12, pp. 1915–1922.)

Treatment of septic shock is multidimensional, with drainage of the septic location, antimicrobial therapy, and cardiovascular support being the three most important factors. A detailed treatise on septic shock is beyond the scope of this manual. The reader is referred to the American Veterinary Medical Association–sponsored *Symposium on Shock* [12]. Table 15–2 summarizes the treatment priorities for this disease. Patient response to therapy is used to change or alter shock treatment.

Septic shock may occur in any septic process when the animal is overwhelmed by infection. Prostatic abscesses, severe necrotizing pancreatitis, peritonitis, severe burns, mastitis, severe biliary-tract infections, and gastric dilation and volvulus are examples. Many gram-negative bacteria produce endotoxins from the lipopolysaccharide portion of their cell membrane. The effects of these endotoxins are multidimensional and may cause many of the pathophysiologic problems associated with septic shock.

Postoperative Concerns

It is unfortunate that many postovariohysterectomy patients are inadequately observed for signs of hemorrhage. Assessment of capillary refill time and mucus membrane colorization are poor criteria for critical evaluation of abdominal blood loss. Often, the problem is noted only after some time has elapsed, or when the animal appears depressed or moribund. Should one observe hemorrhage from the abdominal incision, pale mucus membranes, hypotension, severe depression, or a distended abdomen, the animal should be assessed for evidence of acute blood loss. When in doubt, serial packed cell volume/total solids and systolic blood pressure should be measured. Once abdominal hemorrhage is diagnosed, the patient should be stabilized and returned to the operating room for exploration.

MALE GENITALIA

Surgical procedures in this area are common. Neutering is one of the most frequently performed operations in many practices. In addition, surgery may be performed to treat traumatic injuries, drain abscesses, biopsy and treat cancer, and correct congenital defects.

Orchiectomy

This is one of the most commonly performed surgical procedures. Postoperative concerns include:

1. Hemorrhage. Postoperative hemorrhage can range from minor, with distention of the scrotal sac, to major, life-threatening bleeding from a poorly applied ligature. Hemorrhage may not be evident initially, as the spermatic cord is retracted into the inguinal canal. Patients should be observed regularly for signs of blood loss. We have observed animals with significant blood loss due to ligature failure associated with closed orchiectomy techniques.
2. Bruising and swelling of the scrotum may occur, and this seems to encourage licking by the animal. Licking only exacerbates the problem. At times, scrotal ablation is necessary following hemorrhage and licking-induced scrotal enlargement.
3. Arteriovenous fistula. This rare, postorchiectomy complication has been reported following the procedure [13]. Significant postoperative hemorrhage occurred, and several months later, the fistula developed.

Cryptorchidism

Removal of undescended testes may involve exploration either proximal or distal to the inguinal ring. In cases with testes proximal to the inguinal ring, the abdomen must be entered. Special postoperative concerns include:

1. Hemorrhage. Bleeding may occur because of improper ligation of the spermatic vessels. In cases of intraabdominal testes, it may be occult. Patients should be monitored periodically with appropriate measures.
2. It seems that parapucial and scrotal or inguinal incisions are more apt to cause licking. Elizabethan collars should be used postoperatively.

Vasectomy

Ligation or removal of a portion of the vas deferens rarely is done. It may be performed, however, in certain captive wild animals or domestic pets for special reasons.

Dissection of the spermatic cord and ligation of the vas deferens often produces extensive swelling. If possible, apply cold compresses during recovery from anesthesia, and use an Elizabethan collar during the postsurgical period.

Penile Surgery

By the very nature of the erectile tissue present, hemorrhage often follows penile surgery. Penile procedures include repair of lacerations, correction of urethral prolapse, paraphimosis, repair of congenital abnormalities such as hypospadias, and treatment of malicious injury such as strangulation from a rubber band. Penile urethrostomy may be necessary to remove uroliths lodged at the proximal aspect of the os penis. Postoperative concerns include:

1. Hemorrhage. Bleeding may be intermittent and associated with urination or penile erection. It can be especially troubling following penile urethrostomy, as these wounds often are left open to heal by second intention.
2. Fractures of the os penis are rare. Urethral integrity may be compromised, and catheterization may be necessary. Rarely will callous formation during fracture healing cause urinary obstruction. Fractures with severe penile trauma may necessitate partial amputation of the penis.
3. If the penis has been fractured or the urethral integrity violated, catheterization may be necessary.

Prostate

Surgery of the prostate is done for diagnostic purposes, to resect neoplasia, and to treat or drain abscesses. Surgical access to the prostate is challenging. It often involves splitting the pelvis or removing the pelvic floor for exposure.

Perioperative complications of prostatic abscess drainage include:

Painful caudal abdomen,
Scrotal/prepucial/hindlimb edema,
Hypoproteinemia,
Hypoglycemia,
Anemia,
Sepsis/shock,
Hypokalemia,
Urine leakage,
Urinary incontinence,
Death,
Drain removal by dog,
Arrhythmias,
Recurrent abscess,
Wound infection,
Pneumonia, and
Urine leakage from incision.

Special postoperative concerns include:

1. Urethral catheterization. In cases of total or subtotal prostatectomy, prolonged catheterization may be necessary. It is important to secure the catheter externally to prevent dislodgement, because recatheterization may prove to be very difficult. Use of a closed urinary-drainage system is advised to minimize infection.

2. Sepsis. Prostatic abscesses may result in sepsis. When abscesses are drained, there is significant contamination of the adjacent tissues. Patients treated surgically for abscesses should be monitored carefully for impending signs of sepsis.

3. Drainage. Prostatic abscesses may be drained externally with a Penrose or other drain, or they may be marsupialized. This procedure involves draining prostatic cysts or abscesses percutaneously by suturing the prostatic capsule to the inguinal skin. This allows for the cyst or abscess to be flushed percutaneously and drainage to occur. Immediately following prostatic drainage, complications such as scrotal/ hindlimb edema, sepsis, urine leakage, urinary incontinence, and hypoproteinemia may occur. In 92 dogs treated with Penrose drainage of prostatic abscesses, 19 died or were euthanized during the perioperative period [14]; significant short-term postoperative complications occurred in 72% of cases. This is not a benign procedure, as recurrent urinary tract infection, incontinence, or persistent drainage may occur. In rare instances, herniation of abdominal contents through the defect created in the body wall for marsupialization may occur. It is important to protect the drain so that the patient does not remove it.

Urethrostomy

Urethrostomy is done on the dog and cat primarily to relieve acute urinary obstruction caused by uroliths or neoplasia. These patients may have some degree of postrenal azotemia and hyperkalemia, and they require renal and metabolic assessment before surgery [15]. Complications following urethrostomy include dysuria, pollakiuria, hematuria, and hemorrhage from the surgical site. Recurrent urinary tract infection and stricture formation also may occur. In a follow-up study on cats after perineal urethrostomy [16], 35% had recurrent urinary tract infections. Elizabethan collars are a must to prevent self-mutilation.

REFERENCES

1. Matthews KA, et al: Nephrotoxicity in dogs associated with methoxyfluorane anesthesia and flunixin meglumine analgesia. *Can Vet J* 31:766–771, 1990.
2. Ihle SL, Kostolich M: Acute renal failure associated with contrast medium administration in a dog. *J Am Vet Med Assoc* 199:899–901, 1991.
3. Gahring DR, et al: Comparative renal function studies of nephrotomy closure with and without sutures in dogs. *J Am Vet Med Assoc* 171:537–541, 1977.
4. Greenwood KM, Rawlings CA: Removal of canine renal calculi by pyelolithotomy. *Vet Surg* 10:12–21, 1981.
5. Leveille R: Complications after ultrasound-guided biopsy of abdominal structures in dogs and cats. *J Am Vet Med Assoc* 203:413–415, 1993.
6. McLaughlin MA: Ectopic Ureters—New Concepts in Diagnosis and Surgical Management. *In Publ:* Amer Coll of Veterinary Sciences. ACVS Proceedings, Oct. 24–27, 1993. San Francisco, 1993, 255–257.

7. Stone EA, Mason LK. Surgery of ectopic ureters: types, methods of correction, and postoperative results. *JAAHA* 26:81–88, 1990.
8. Selcer RA: Urinary tract trauma associated with pelvic trauma. *JAAHA* 18:785–793, 1982.
9. Burrows CF, Bonee KC: Metabolic changes due to experimentally induced rupture of the canine urinary bladder. *Am J Vet Res* 35:1083–1088, 1974.
10. Wheaton LG, et al: Results and complications of surgical treatment of pyometra. *JAAHA* 25:563–568, 1989.
11. Kenney KS, et al: Pyometra in cats: 183 cases (1979–1984). *J Am Vet Med Assoc* 191: 1130, 1987.
12. Haskins SC: Management of septic shock: symposia. *J Am Vet Med Assoc* 200: 1915–1922, 1992.
13. Aiken SW: Acquired arteriovenous fistula secondary to castration in the dog. *J Am Vet Med Assoc* 202:965–967, 1993.
14. Mullen HS, Mathiesen DT, Scarelli TD: Results of surgery and postoperative complications in 92 dogs treated for prostatic abscessation by a multiple Penrose drain technique. *JAAHA* 26:369–379, 1990.
15. Gregory CR, Vasseur PB: Long term examination of cats with perineal urethrostomy. *Vet Surg* 12:210–212, 1983.
16. Hosgood G, Hedlund CS: Perineal urethrostomy in cats. *Comp Cont Ed Pract Vet* 14: 1195–1205, 1992.

16

Cardiac Procedures

Cardiac procedures often are referred to specialized centers that possess cardiopulmonary-bypass equipment, invasive cardiovascular monitors, specialized diagnostic equipment, and staff with specialized training. There are some procedures such as patent ductus arteriosus, pacemaker placement, vascular ring anomalies, and resection of atrial tumors that do not require pulmonary bypass. By their nature, cardiac procedures do require a thoracotomy. This may be accomplished via an intracostal approach, mediastinostomy, a transthoracic approach, or a laparotomy followed by diaphragmatic incision.

Only the most common operative cardiovascular procedures are covered here. In the event a more complicated procedure involving cardiac standstill using hypothermia or cardiopulmonary bypass is anticipated, a detailed postoperative plan should be developed before surgery. Aortic stenosis, tetralogy of Fallot, atrial and ventricular septal defects, as well as mitral and tricuspid defects, require cardiopulmonary bypass assistance. These procedures need specialized equipment and personnel and rarely are performed in the average surgical practice.

GENERAL POSTOPERATIVE CONCERNS

Restoration of Pleural Space

During any thoracotomy, it is mandatory to remove air and/or fluid from the pleural space (see Chapter V). Ideally, this is achieved with low-pressure, intermittent suction via a sealed water bottle or commercially available device. If possible, one should avoid periodic pleural-space evacuation with a syringe, because it is possible to suck the lung over the opening in the tube and get a false sense of negative pressure. Heimlich valves are of no use during pleural-space evacuation in small animals and should not be used. These patients should be monitored with periodic radiographs, thoracic auscultation, measurement of fluid return, pulse oximetry, blood-gas analysis, and measurement of blood or central venous system pressure as the situation dictates.

Blood Loss

Closed pleural-space drainage can provide an accurate assessment of postoperative blood loss. Coupled with intraoperative blood losses, this can be used to determine the need for packed red blood cells or volume replacement. Packed cell volume, total solids, blood pressure, and pulse oximetry can be important values to monitor postsurgically. Autotransfusion is greatly facilitated when closed pleural-space drainage is used (see Chapter X).

Cardiac Arrhythmias and Overload

During procedures involving the myocardium when ligation of vessels is done or with some valvular reconstructions, arrhythmias may occur. Periodic electrocardiographic or telemetric monitoring can be useful, as can central venous pressure, blood-gas analysis, and cardiac catheterization.

PATENT DUCTUS ARTERIOSUS

Patent ductus arteriosus (PDA) is the most common congenital cardiac disorder of the dog. The ductus arteriosus normally shunts blood from the pulmonary artery and aorta in the fetus. Failure of closure allows abnormal shunting of high-pressure aortic blood into the pulmonary artery; this produces pulmonary hypertension and pulmonary edema. A characteristic, continuous or machine-like murmur is auscultated on both sides of the hemithorax. Definitive diagnosis includes plain radiographs, ultrasound, and occasionally, cardiac catheterization to quantitate intracardiac pressure differentials.

Treatment for PDA is surgery. The procedure is done via a left-sided thoracotomy and involves ligating the shunt between the aorta and pulmonary artery. It is important to ascertain that a left-to-right shunt exists before surgery. As pulmonary hypertension persists, permanent pulmonary changes may reverse the shunting to right-to-left, and these patients do not benefit from surgical ligation. Correction of PDA in experienced hands is a relatively safe procedure. In 201 cases of surgically corrected PDA [1], 89% were alive and normal at 1-month following surgery. Besides hemorrhage, postoperative complications include cardiac arrest, iatrogenic lung trauma, ventricular arrhythmias, sepsis, and recanalization of the ductus.

Special postoperative concerns include:

1. Thoracotomy. Because this procedure is done via a left thoracotomy, principles of chest tube management are followed here (see Chapter VII).

2. Hemorrhage. In very short shunts, it is possible to tear the ductus near the aorta, especially as dissection is carried around the shunt. Hemorrhage must be controlled in the operating room, but the patient may come to the recovery area in need of additional cardiovascular support. Whole-blood replacement, packed red blood cells, and fluid volume replacement may be needed. In this case, parameters to monitor blood loss and hypotension are needed. These include packed cell volume/total solids, blood pressure, pulse oximetry, blood-gas analysis, and blood pressure monitoring.

PACEMAKER IMPLANTATION

Complete heart block can be treated surgically by implanting a unipolar fixed-rate or demand-rate pacemaker (Fig. 16–1). Animals with complete heart block are

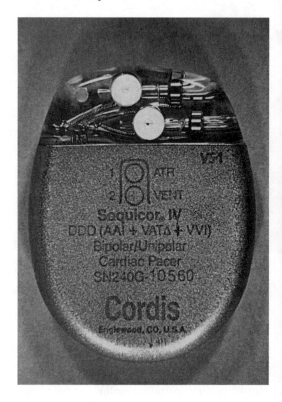

Fig. 16–1. A demand-rate pacemaker ready for implantation. (Courtesy of Peter Schwarz, DVM.)

critically ill and often have coexisting metabolic diseases, such as diabetes or renal compromise. Often, a transvenous pacemaker is introduced into the jugular vein for temporary cardiac pacing. Once a normal heart rate is established, the animal can be anesthetized in the usual way. A left-lateral thoracotomy or transdiaphragmatic approach via an abdominal incision is used to implant the pacemaker electrode. Following incision of the pericardium, the screw electrode is attached to the left, ventricular apex. The electrode wires are tunneled percutaneously, and the battery pack is implanted in the abdominal cavity.

Special postoperative concerns include:

1. Thoracotomy management (see Chapter VII).
2. Infection. While usually not evident in the first 1 to 2 days following implantation, infections may require removal of the pacemaker. Often, prophylactic antibiotics are used and continued for several days following surgery.
3. Seromas associated with implantation of the battery pack may develop. They should be aspirated and the contents submitted for culture and susceptibility testing.
4. Wire or electrode displacement. This is an infrequent complication but usually requires reoperation for repair.

PERICARDECTOMY

Persistent pericardial effusion may produce significant cardiac tamponade. When periodic pericardiocentesis fails, pericardectomy is advised. In animals receiving a pericardectomy for benign pericardial effusion, 50% have a favorable outcome [2]. The pericardium is approached via a left-lateral thoracotomy or transdiaphragmatic approach via an abdominal incision, and as much of the pericardium is removed as possible.

Special postoperative concerns include:

1. Thoracotomy management (see Chapter VII).
2. Hemorrhage. In many instances, the pericardium is very thickened and contains reactive granulation tissue. Intrapleural hemorrhage can be measured via chest-tube output. If significant bleeding occurs, hemodynamic support measures such as autotransfusion, administration of packed red blood cells, or whole blood may be indicated.

CARDIAC TUMORS

Hemangiosarcomas of the right atria are common in animals prone to hemangiosarcoma (e.g., German Shepherds), and these tumors produce pericardial effusion and cardiac tamponade. Isolated hemangiosarcomas may be surgically excised, but the long-term prognosis is poor. A left-lateral thoracotomy is performed, and following excision of the pericardium, the right atrial tumor is isolated and most often excised with an automatic stapling device.

Special postoperative concerns include:

1. Thoracotomy management (see Chapter VII).
2. Hemorrhage. Provided that no technical failure occurs with the stapling device, there is little intrapleural hemorrhage. Careful observation of chest-tube drainage can help to rule out significant hemorrhage.

VASCULAR RING ANOMALIES

Vascular ring anomalies associated with the aortic arch are common in the dog and cat. A persistent right aortic arch is most common and causes compromise of the esophagus (Fig. 16–2). Most animals present with a history of regurgitation. Both plain and contrast radiography and/or ultrasound are used to demonstrate the vascular ring anomaly. A left-lateral thoracotomy is used to approach and ligate the ligamentus arteriosum.

Special postoperative concerns include:

1. Thoracotomy and chest-tube management.
2. Aspiration pneumonia. These patients have a dilated and poorly functioning esophagus. There often is putrid food trapped cranial to the obstruction. Ideally, this material has been evacuated before surgery. It is advisable to suction the pharynx

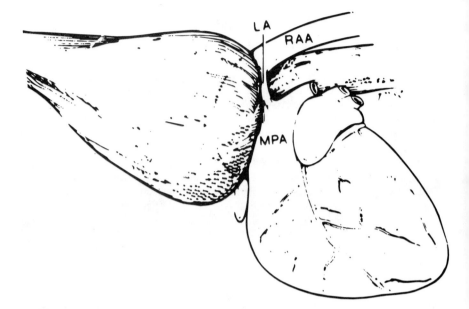

Fig. 16–2. Persistent right aortic arch (RAA) and esophageal compromise. (Slatter, D.: Textbook of Small Animal Surgery. Philadelphia, W.B. Saunders, 1993, p. 683.)

and esophagus before tracheal extubation. While the recovering patient is in lateral recumbency, fluids may ascend the esophagus and be aspirated. Delay tracheal extubation until normal reflexes are present; this can minimize aspiration. Should significant aspiration occur, especially if large food particles are present, the patient should be reanesthetized and the tracheobronchial tree thoroughly suctioned of foreign material. Broad-spectrum antimicrobial therapy should begin immediately.

REFERENCES

1. Birchard SJ, Bonagura JD, Fingland RB: Results of ligation of PDA in dogs: 201 cases (1969–1988). *J Am Vet Med Assoc* 196:2011–2013, 1990.
2. Eyster GE, Jaber CE, Probst M: Cardiac disorders. *In* Slatter D, editor. Textbook of Small Animal Surgery. Philadelphia, 1993, WB Saunders, pp. 856–889.

17

Respiratory Procedures

Upper respiratory surgery may be done to correct anatomic defects such as stenotic nares and elongated soft palate, to perform biopsy, and to treat laryngeal disease or neoplasia. Of special concern are patients with existing airway disease such as occurs in brachycephalic breeds, animals with airway obstruction from tumors or abscess, and those with chronic or persistent cardiovascular disease.

In emergent situations or as a presurgical procedure, tracheostomy may be necessary. Tracheostomy is not a benign procedure, and it requires considerable postoperative care. The suggested protocol for the management of tracheostomy should include:

1. Lavage and suction. One should inject 1 to 5 mL of PSS into the tracheostomy orifice to moisturize the trachea and help mobilize mucus. Using a flexible tube, the orifice and tube should be suctioned (Fig. 17–1).
2. Maintenance of tube patency. Using the stylet (Fig. 17–2), the tube should be cleaned to prevent mucus from accumulating in the opening of the tracheostomy tube.
3. The tracheostomy tube should be anchored firmly to adjacent soft tissue to prevent dislodgement (Fig. 17–3).
4. Careful observation is a must to ensure that the orifice does not become occluded by bedding, bandages, or skin folds of the neck.
5. Patients with tracheostomy tubes should be kept in the intensive care unit for continuous monitoring.

After soft-palate resection or surgery of the larynx, nasopharyngeal and laryngeal tissues may become edematous and obstruct airflow. Pulse oximetry, auscultation, and blood-gas analysis may be helpful parameters to monitor. If airway obstruction is caused by edema, reintubation or tracheostomy may be necessary. Furosemide (Hoechst-Roussel, Somerville, N.J.) (2–4 mg/kg body weight) and/or methylprednisolone (0.25 mg/kg) also may be indicated.

Brachycephalic breeds always have some degree of persistent airway obstruction. Their postsurgical management needs special concern and includes:

1. An in-circuit humidifier for inhalation anesthesia helps to prevent drying of the airway.

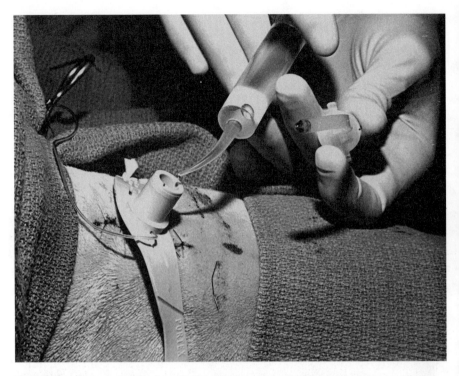

Fig. 17–1. Three to 5 mL of sterile saline injected into the tracheostomy stoma. (Courtesy of David M. Ennis, DVM.)

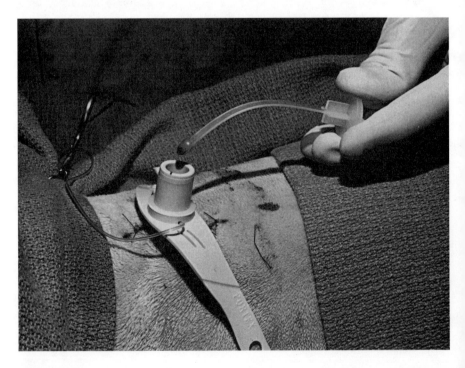

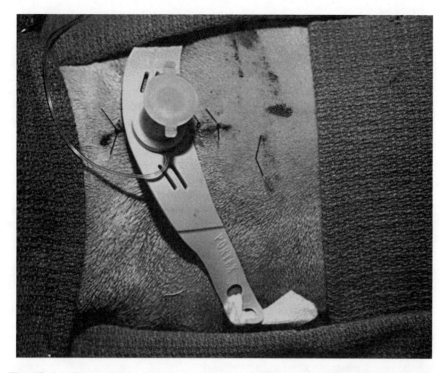

Fig. 17–3. The tracheostomy tube is securely bandaged or sutured to the adjacent skin. (Courtesy of David M. Ennis, DVM.)

2. An open intravenous line is mandatory for anesthesia in any brachycephalic breed.
3. After the procedure is finished, prolong extubation until the patient is sternally recumbent. Fentanyl or butorphanol can be given 0.11 to 0.15 mL/kg or 8 to 1.2 mg/kg, respectively, to provide relaxation and recovery after surgery. With the use of one of these drugs, the endotracheal tube can be left in until recovery from the anesthesia is complete.
4. The anesthetist must sit with the patient to manage the tube and monitor recovery. In some instances, recovery of a brachycephalic breed may take hours.
5. Hyperthermia may be problematic if severe tachypnea and dyspnea continue untreated.
6. Pulse oximetry is a useful, noninvasive way to monitor oxygen saturation in these breeds.
7. It may be advisable to administer supplemental oxygen via a nasal oxygen catheter. Ideally, the catheter is placed before anesthetic recovery and used during the postanesthetic recovery.

Fig. 17–2. The stylet is quickly introduced and removed to clear the tube of mucus. (Courtesy of David M. Ennis, DVM.)

LARYNGEAL PARALYSIS

Laryngeal paralysis is an acquired disease of older, large-breed dogs, and it is characterized by an inability to abduct the arytenoid cartilage during inspiration. Respiratory stridor and compromise occur, especially with exercise. In some patients, signs of generalized neurologic disease may exist. The problem most often is unilateral. There are three commonly performed procedures to treat this problem. Bilateral vocal chordectomy and partial laryngectomy (Fig. 17–4) is performed per os using elongated instruments. A presurgical tracheostomy often is recommended, and hemorrhage from the procedure is controlled either with tamponade or electrosurgical coagulation.

Modified laryngeal castellation involves approaching the larynx ventrally and incising the thyroid cartilage in a stepwise fashion (Fig. 17–5). It is sutured so that the ventral aspect of the thyroid cartilage is wedged open. Presurgical placement of a tracheostomy tube usually is advised and subsequently is removed following surgery and anesthetic recovery.

Unilateral arytenoid cartilage lateralization is performed via a lateral approach to the larynx. This procedure lateralizes the arytenoid (Fig. 17–6) cartilage by suturing it either to the thyroid or cricoid cartilage. If this procedure is performed bilaterally, there is some risk of aspiration pneumonia developing as a postsurgical complication. The endotracheal tube should remain in place until protective pharyngeal reflexes are regained.

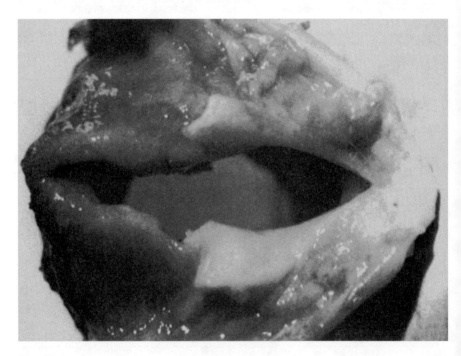

Fig. 17–4. A partial laryngectomy is performed to alleviate dyspnea caused by laryngeal paralysis. (Veterinary Surgery, Vol. 12(4), p. 198.)

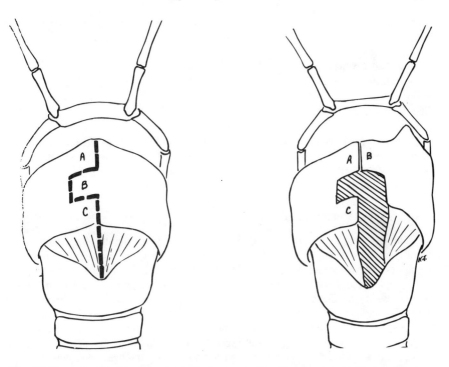

Fig. 17–5. A modified laryngeal castellation can help to increase laryngeal circumference. (Slatter, D.: Textbook of Small Animal Surgery. Philadelphia, W.B. Saunders, 1993, p. 682.)

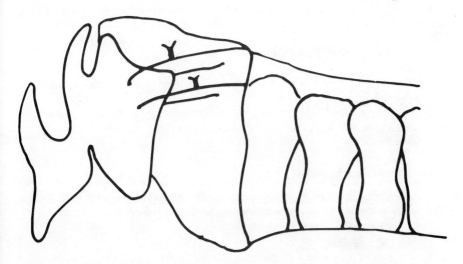

Fig. 17–6. The arytenoid cartilage is sutured to secure it more laterally. (With permission from Slatter, D.: Textbook of Small Animal Surgery. Philadelphia, W.B. Saunders, 1993, p. 682.)

Surgery distal to the larynx may be performed to remove growths or foreign bodies, correct collapsing airways, repair traumatic injury, and diagnose and treat cancer. In general, two major concerns exist: tracheostomy placement and care if needed, and restoration of pleural space.

TRACHEAL SURGERY

The trachea may be operated on to correct flaccid tracheal rings, repair lacerations, remove foreign bodies and tumors, and rarely, resect fistulae. A permanent or temporary tracheostomy may be done and up to four tracheal rings resected with the severed ends anastomosed.

Surgery for Collapsing Trachea

Collapsing trachea is a disease of the tracheal cartilage whereby the degenerative changes in the cartilaginous rings cause the tracheal rings to lose their strength and durability. The trachea cannot maintain normal conformation during the respiratory cycle, and dorsoventral collapse occurs. Collapsing trachea is a form of airway obstruction most common in middle- to older-aged, small dogs. It is treated both medically and surgically. Surgery is performed to stent the tracheal rings with prosthetic tracheal implants; the implants are made by cutting polypropylene syringe cases into cylinders of the appropriate size. Following production of the prostheses, they are sterilized and implanted around the collapsing trachee.

Acute respiratory distress is a special postoperative concern. Some degree of airway obstruction and inflammation may persist. Often, there is significant coughing that can exacerbate tracheal irritation. Supplemental O_2 via a nasal catheter, an O_2 cage, supplemental sedatives (e.g., acepromazine), or a bronchodilator (e.g., aminophylline) may be given. Antibiotic therapy is indicated if bacterial tracheitis is present. Ideally, recovery from anesthesia should begin in a quiet, nonstressful environment.

Special postoperative concerns include:

1. Airway patency. It is vital that the airways be free of blood, mucus, and tissue obstruction.
2. Air leakage. It is important to have an airtight repair or tracheal anastomosis to prevent subcutaneous leakage and emphysema, pneumomediastinum, or pneumothorax.

Permanent Tracheostomy

This procedure is done to bypass permanently the larynx and proximal trachea. The stoma is created in the midcervical region (Fig. 17–7).

Special postoperative concerns include:

1. The patient will have a tracheostomy tube in place; as recovery occurs, it is removed. It is advisable to place a small amount of triple-antibiotic ointment around the skin, tracheal mucosa, and site.
2. The stoma site must be kept free of obstruction and be suctioned periodically.

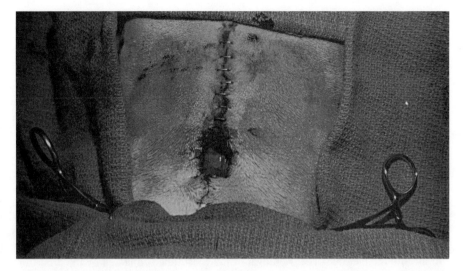

Fig. 17–7. A permanent tracheostomy is done by suturing the sternothyroid muscle to its dorsal and lateral edges. Several tracheal rings are partially removed and the skin sutured to the tracheal mucosa. (Courtesy of David M. Ennis, DVM.)

3. Humidification of ambient air might be helpful for the first several days following surgery.

THORACIC SURGERY

Thoracic surgery is performed to gain access to the thoracic pleural space, heart, lungs, and mediastinum. Diseases of the lungs requiring surgery include neoplasia, lung-lobe torsion, abscesses, bullae causing pneumothorax, lacerations, or broncho-esophageal fistulas. The mediastinum is the space between the two hemithoraces, and it contains the heart and great vessels, trachea, esophagus, thymus, lymph nodes, and various nerves [1]. Given the many structures in the chest, specific postoperative concerns may be reflected by the organs or tissues involved. In general, there are a group of concerns regarding thoracotomy that deserve emphasis. These include special analgesia needs, hypoventilation, care and integrity of the chest tube, hypoxemia, hypothermia, acid–base disorders, and hypotension.

Postoperative concerns include:

1. Postoperative analgesia. Thoracotomy is associated with significant postoperative pain, and several special analgesic methods deserve mentioning. Intercostal nerve blocks can be performed either during or immediately after surgery. If bupivacaine is used, analgesia may last 4 to 6 hours. Intrapleural analgesia may be produced by instilling lidocaine or bupivacaine into the pleural space following pleural closure. These special analgesic methods may be combined with conventional techniques to provide a smooth, less painful recovery (see Chapter IV).

2. Care of the chest tube. Placement of one or more tubes into the pleural space is mandatory before thoracic closure. The tube size should approximate the diameter of the mainstem bronchus [2]; for example:

Cats and dogs <7 kg	14–16 Fr
Dogs 7–15 kg	18–22 Fr
Dogs 16–30 kg	22–28 Fr
Dogs >30 kg	28–36 Fr

The chest tube must be secured to the skin to ensure against its dislodgment (Fig. 17–8). It is connected via tubing to a two- or three-bottle suction apparatus. Alternatively, a commercial pleural evacuation system [*DeKnatel* (Division of Pfizer Hosp. Products Group Inc.) Floral Park, N.Y.] (Pleurvac) may be used. The first bottle to which the chest tube is connected collects air or fluid from the pleural space; this bottle is then connected to a second bottle containing water with the suction-tubing set below the surface of the water. The water acts as a seal against the movement of air into the pleural space. Removal of the chest tube is dictated by the procedure and integrity of the pleural space. Hypoventilation and hypoxemia following thoracic surgery most often result from continuing air leaks and often can be managed effectively with appropriate chest-tube drainage. Contents from the chest tube mirror the activity of the pleural space and can be used to monitor progress. For example, continued hemorrhage will be evident in the chest bottles, as will continued leakage of air.

3. Hypothermia can be a significant postsurgical problem in open-chest procedures. Prompt recognition and rewarming of the animal with warm-water blankets or warm blankets is important during recovery. Using an intravenous fluid warmer (Fig. 17–9) or warm fluids also can be beneficial.

4. Hypoventilation. Using a Wright's respirometer, tidal volume can be measured or end-tidal carbon dioxide determined to access ventilation. A tidal volume less than 10 mL/kg or end-tidal CO_2 greater than 55 mm Hg suggests hypoventilation.

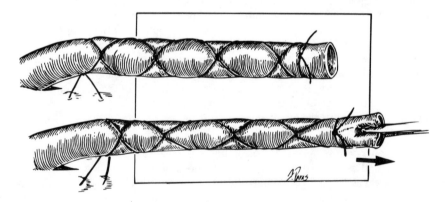

Fig. 17–8. The chest tube is secured to the skin with the chinese finger-trap method, then bandaged to keep it secure. (Smeak, D.D.: Chinese finger trap suture technique for fastening tubes and catheters. JAAHA 26:215, 1990.)

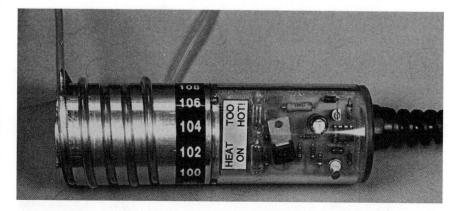

Fig. 17–9. This device helps to warm intravenous fluids before administration to minimize fluid-induced hypothermia. (Courtesy of David M. Ennis, DVM.)

This problem may result from air or fluid in the pleural space or drug-related respiratory depression, and it should be treated accordingly.

5. Hypoxemia most often is caused by ventilation–perfusion mismatch. Significant pulmonary congestion may be present in the down lung after prolonged lateral recumbency. Appropriate ventilation, supplemental O_2, and positive end-expiratory pressure are recommended.

REFERENCES

1. Moon M: Radiology of the mediastinum and pleural space. *In* Proceedings, ACVS, 1993, Vet. Symp., San Francisco, pp. 202–204.
2. Boothe HW: Pleural effusion: diagnosis and therapy. *In* Proceedings, ACVS, 1993, San Francisco, CA., pp. 211–213.

18

Laparoscopic Abdominal Surgery

Laparoscopy is in its infancy in clinical veterinary surgery, but it is widely used on dogs and pigs for teaching and research. General anesthesia is required, and the abdominal cavity is distended with carbon dioxide or nitrous oxide. A laparoscope varying in diameter from 2 to 10 mm is introduced into the distended abdomen to allow visualization. Additional abdominal portals are established through stab incisions to allow the introduction of instruments. To better understand this new technology, a more detailed description of the equipment and procedures is required.

EQUIPMENT

Rigid Endoscopes

Rigid endoscopes vary in diameter, with 8 or 10 mm being the most popular. Good depth of field and magnification is provided by 0° or forward-viewing 30° scopes (Fig. 18–1).

Insufflator

The operative field and abdominal cavity are exposed by gas insufflation with CO_2 (Fig. 18–2). Creation of a pneumoperitoneum allows visualization and manipulation of the abdominal contents. A high-flow insufflator delivering 8 to 10 L/min can automatically maintain a constant intraabdominal pressure of between 12 to 15 mm Hg.

Light Source

A high-intensity light source is used to illuminate the surgical field. It is supplied to the laparoscope via glass fibers.

Video Monitors and Camera

Video cameras are designed to fit the laparoscope to allow visualization of the procedure, which is displayed on a high-resolution monitor (Fig. 18–3). Modern video cameras are very small and offer single- or three-chip digital signal processing, and are designed to be cold sterilized (i.e., submersion) or gas sterilized.

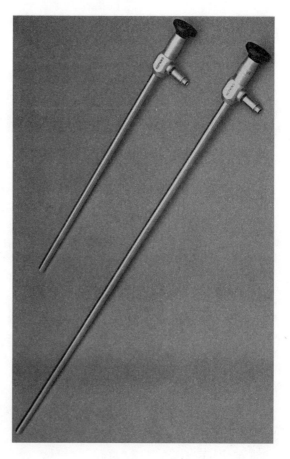

Fig. 18–1. A 30° forward-viewing laparoscope. (Courtesy of Karl Storz.)

Operating and Equipment Portals

Additional access to the abdomen is gained via portals that are placed advantageous to the procedure. Following insufflation, operating portals are trocared, and both instruments and operative specimens can be managed through the sealed portal (Fig. 18–4).

SPECIAL POSTOPERATIVE CONCERNS

Given the broad gamut of procedures currently performed, the list of potential problems parallels these procedures.

Trocar Placement

The initial trocar placement to allow for insertion of the laparoscope may injure or lacerate the adjacent loops of bowel, spleen, liver, or major blood vessels. This

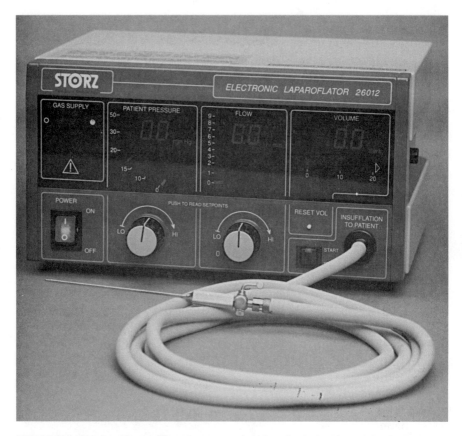

Fig. 18–2.   This insufflator allows the operator to select the desired intraabdominal pressure and monitor it. (Courtesy of Karl Storz.)

potential is minimized by using a Verres needle to create a mild pneumoperitoneum before insertion of the laparoscope. Insertion of the Verres needle for initial insufflation or trocar placement also may injure the adjacent loops of bowel, spleen, liver, or major retroperitoneal vessels. The Verres needle is designed to reduce the risk of visceral injury, as it has an inner, spring-loaded, blunt stylet that protects the viscera from the sharp outer sheath after entry into the peritoneal cavity. Viscera that are adhesed to the ventral abdominal wall still may be perforated or lacerated. Care should be exercised when significant peritoneal adhesions are suspected or the animal has had prior abdominal surgery.

In humans, the incidence of visceral injury following Verres needle or trocar insertion varies from 0.05% to 2.00% [1]. Injury to major retroperitoneal vessels occurs in 0.05% of cases [2]. Following placement of the Verres needle, a mild pneumoperitoneum is created, and the laparoscope with cannula and trocar are inserted. Hernia development at the insertion site occurs in 0.1% to 0.3% of cases [3].

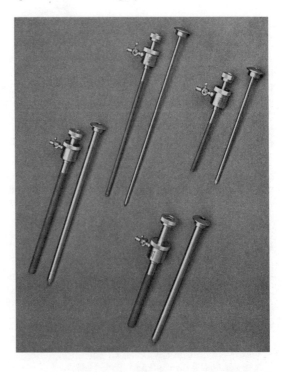

Fig. 18–3. The operating portal allows instruments to be introduced near the operative field. More than one portal may be necessary in complex laparoscopic procedures. (Courtesy of Karl Storz.)

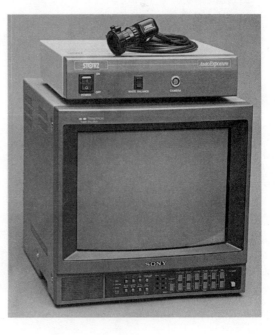

Fig. 18–4. A high-resolution, three-chip video camera adaptable to the laparoscope. (Courtesy of Karl Storz.)

Insufflation

Carbon dioxide is the gas most commonly used to distend the abdomen. It is possible to create CO_2-induced acid–base disturbances with this gas. In addition, the induced pneumoperitoneum greatly decreases tidal volume, and mechanical ventilation during the procedure therefore is advisable. It is possible to create a pneumothorax with proximal dissection of the abdominal esophagus, and insufflation can be problematic in patients with a torn diaphragm. A fatal case of air embolism associated with nitrogen insufflation administered via a Verres needle in the left flank has been documented [4].

Cardiac arrhythmias are common when CO_2 is used for abdominal insufflation [5]. They most commonly are ventricular extrasystoles, but vagal stimulation during insufflation may produce a bradycardia. Animals recovering from abdominal laparoscopy should be monitored postoperatively for arrhythmias.

REFERENCES

1. Kone MG, Kreigs GJ: Complications of diagnostic laparoscopy in Dallas: a 7-year prospective study. *Gastrointestinal Endoscopy* 30:237–240, 1984.
2. Dezeil DJ, et al: Complications of laparoscopic cholecystectomy: results of a national survey of 4,292 hospitals and analysis of 77,604 cases. *Am J Surg* 165:9–14, 1993.
3. Peters JH, et al: Complications of laparoscopic cholecystectomy. *Surgery* 110:769–778, 1991.
4. Gilroy BA, Anson LW: Fatal air embolism during anesthesia for laparoscopy in a dog. *J Am Vet Med Assoc* 190:552–554, 1987.
5. Crist DW, Gadacz TR: Complications of laparoscopic surgery. *Surg Clin North Am* 73: 265–288, 1993.

19

Ophthalmic Surgery

TODD HAMMOND, DVM

Ophthalmic surgeries are commonly performed, and they range from repair of minor lid deformities to complex intraocular procedures [1]. Meticulous attention to detail is necessary for success, because minor postoperative problems can compromise operative success and jeopardize vision.

Corticosteroids commonly are used both pre- and postoperatively to reduce inflammation. By virtue of their antiprostaglandin action, corticosteroids reduce inflammatory protein leakage into the aqueous humor. Use of corticosteroids in the perioperative period slow wound healing and reduce resistance to disease. Topical corticosteroids can or are able to (not common occurrence) suppress adrenocorticotropic-hormone release and lower serum-cortisol levels [2]. These effects should be acknowledged and taken into account postoperatively.

Nonsteroidal anti-inflammatory drugs (NSAIDs) often are used to provide analgesia and to reduce inflammation (see Chapter VI). Antibiotics are routinely used as topical preparations, incorporated into lavage solutions, and administered systemically.

GENERAL PRINCIPLES OF POSTOPERATIVE CARE FOR OPHTHALMIC PATIENTS

General principles of postoperative care for these patients include:

1. On presentation to the recovery area, make sure that the operative site is clean and no evidence of "clipper burn" or contact dermatitis is evident. If present, these problems will cause the eye to be more painful and possibly subject to self-mutilation.

2. Continue or institute drug therapy. Mannitol may be administered to reduce intraocular pressure. Corticosteroids, NSAIDs, antibiotics, and cycloplegics may be prescribed by the ophthalmic surgeon.

3. Take proactive measures to prevent self-mutilation. In general, Elizabethan collars are recommended for all external ophthalmic procedures. In addition, bandaging the dewclaws and/or the front limbs may be routine (Fig. 19–1). In severe cases, tranquilization (acepromazine, 0.025–0.20 mg/kg body weight intravenously; or diazepam, 0.2–0.6 mg/kg intravenously) may be necessary.

4. Proactive pain control is advisable. Cycloplegics may be advisable for anterior-segment lesions, while systemic analgesics routinely are used in the perioperative period (see Chapter VI).

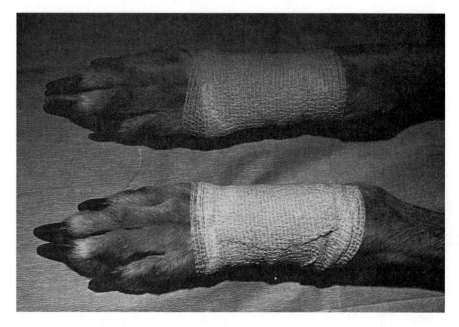

Fig. 19–1.   This patient's front dewclaws have been bandaged to prevent ocular self-mutilation. (Courtesy of David M. Ennis, DVM.)

EYELID SURGERY

Surgery on the eyelids is performed to repair lacerations, resect eyelid tumors, and correct congenital lid defects. Special postoperative concerns include:

1. Routine use of an Elizabethan collar is recommended to prevent self-mutilation and wound disruption.
2. Warm compresses are applied as needed to clean the orbital fissure–periorbital area.
3. Topical or systemic antibiotics may be used following extensive lid reconstructions. NSAIDs may be used to minimize postoperative inflammation.
4. Immediate lid swelling follows cryosurgical procedures and should last from 36 to 72 hours.
5. A temporary tarsorrhaphy may be performed to protect the cornea after eyelid reconstruction.

CORNEAL SURGERY

Corneal surgery is performed to repair lacerations, remove inflammatory tissue, and repair and/or support ulcers and desmetoceles. Special postoperative concerns include:

1. Use of an Elizabethan collar is routine.
2. Topical administration of antibiotics, cycloplegics, and anti-inflammatory steroids and nonsteroidal drugs is routine. Scheduled administration of these drugs should begin and continue in the recovery area. Subcompartmental injections of these drugs may be given postoperatively, ideally while the patient is anesthetized (Fig. 19–2).
3. Corneal contact lenses or collagen shields may be used to protect the cornea (Fig. 19–3).
4. A temporary tarsorrhaphy may be performed to protect the cornea (Fig. 19–4), or a third-eyelid flap may be used.

THIRD EYELID SURGERY

The third eyelid is a triangular structure arising from the medial canthus. Surgery is done to treat prolapse either by replacement or glandular excision. Special concerns include:

1. Elizabethan collars often are unnecessary.
2. Warm compresses are used to clean the eyelids and periorbital tissue.

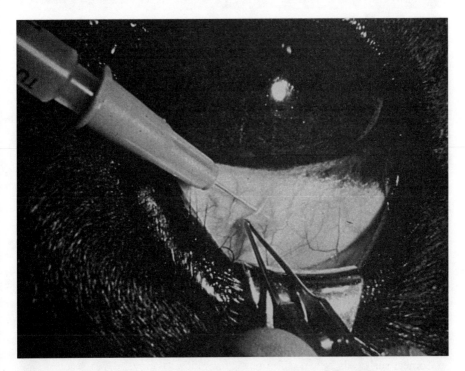

Fig. 19–2. A subconjunctival injection of prednisolone. (Courtesy of Todd Hammond, DVM.)

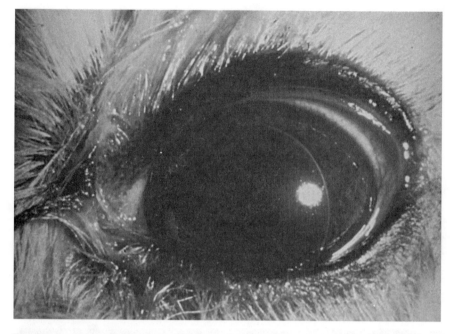

Fig. 19–3.   This collagen shield will protect the corneal laceration while it heals. (Courtesy of Todd Hammond, DVM.)

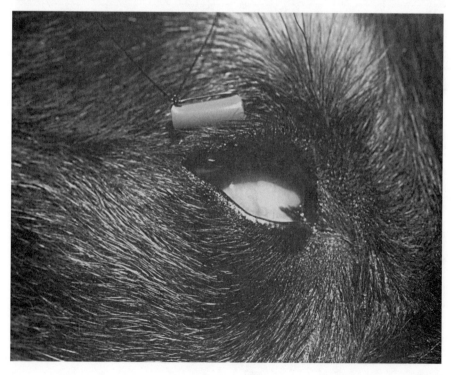

3. Topical antibiotics are routinely administered (triple ophthalmic ointment: 4-mm bead to the affected eye every 6 hours).

INTRAOCULAR SURGERY

Intraocular surgery is performed to remove cataracts, treat lens luxations, treat iris prolapse, and remove intraocular foreign bodies. Special concerns include:

1. The patient is positioned with the head higher than the body during recovery to prevent retinal separation or detachment.

2. An Elizabethan collar can be used to prevent self-mutilation, but this often is unnecessary.

3. Topical antibiotics, cycloplegics, and anti-inflammatory drugs are used routinely following surgery.

4. Antibiotics and anti-inflammatory agents may be given either systemically or subconjunctivally.

5. The patient should be monitored for signs of increased intraocular pressure. The eye can be palpated carefully for increased pressure. Tonometry with a Schiøtz tonometer is more reliable than digital tonometry. Other external signs include vascular injection, pupillary dilation, and corneal edema. Methazolamide (Lederle; Pearl River, N.Y.) 1 to 2 mg/kg twice daily for 48 hours and then 0.5 to 1.0 mg/kg to effect (most effective in small animals <30 lbs), or Dichlorphenamide (Merck-Sharp-Dohme, West Point, PA) 2 to 4 mg/kg orally two or three times a day, are given to reduce intraocular pressure. Intravenous acetazolamide (Lederle, Carolina, Puerto Rico) may be given in emergent situations.

6. Postoperative analgesia and sedation is helpful. Excessive barking or other activity may cause retinal separation following removal of cataract.

7. Prevent increases in abdominal pressure from retching, vomiting, or excessive coughing. Delayed feeding and use of antiemetics (metoclopromide, 0.1–0.5 mg/kg intramuscularly or orally) and antitussives (Butorphanol tartrate, 0.50–0.12 mg/kg orally twice daily) are recommended should these problems arise.

8. If possible, routinely measure systemic blood pressure to detect hypertension and avoid overhydration with intraoperative fluids.

9. Diabetic patients recovering from cataract surgery should have routine monitoring of blood-glucose levels.

GLAUCOMA

Glaucoma is evidenced by increases in intraocular pressure (i.e., >27 to 30 mm Hg) [3] and has many causes. Glaucoma can cause permanent destruction of optic-nerve fiber and frequently is encountered in dogs. The Cocker spaniel, Bouvier des Flandres, Basset hound, Chow-chow, Samoyed, Beagle, and Toy poodle are breeds with a high incidence of glaucoma.

Fig. 19–4. Temporary tarsorrhaphy or application of a third-eyelid flap can provide corneal protection. (Courtesy of David M. Ennis, DVM.)

Surgical treatment of glaucoma may include cryosurgery, placement of a glaucoma shunt valve and an intrascleral prosthesis, and chemical ablation of the ciliary body. Special postoperative concerns include:

1. Routine use of an Elizabethan collar is recommended.
2. Monitor intraocular pressure for 72 hours after surgery. Visible signs of a nonresponsive, dilated pupil; cloudy cornea; or intraocular hemorrhage should be reported immediately. Measurements with a mechanical Schiøtz tonometer or Tono-pen applanation tonometer (Oculab, Glenside, Calif.) should be done at regular intervals.
3. Cryosurgery produces intense chemosis of the conjunctiva, and systemic anti-inflammatory drugs are used postoperatively.
4. A tarsorrhaphy is used routinely with some glaucoma procedures (e.g., intrascleral prosthesis).
5. In chemical ablation of the ciliary body, there is an intense conjunctival scleral reaction for 72 hours. All systemic and topical medications used to control intraocular pressure can stop at the time of surgery.
6. Avoid leashes around the neck following cyclocryosurgery and glaucoma shunt-valve procedures, because sudden increases in blood pressure may cause retinal detachment.

RETINAL PROCEDURES

Retinal procedures include globe exenteration, placement of orbital prostheses, drainage of retroorbital abscesses, and exploration of the orbit for foreign bodies and tumors. Special postoperative concerns include:

1. Use of an Elizabethan collar should be considered only with orbital exploration.
2. Routine use of temporary tarsorrhaphy to protect the cornea.
3. Systemic antibiotics are used following drainage of retroorbital abscesses and prosthetic placement.
4. Systemic NSAIDs are useful for all orbital procedures (see Chapter VI).
5. With orbital prostheses, expect a serous nasal discharge for 48 to 72 hours following surgery.

REFERENCES

1. Slatter D: Eye and adnexa. *In* Slatter D, editor. Textbook of Small Animal Surgery. Philadelphia, 1993, WB Saunders, pp. 1142–1156.
2. Roberts SM, et al: Effect of ophthalmic prednisilone on the canine adrenal gland and hepatic function. *Am J Vet Res* 45:1711–1714, 1984.
3. Lonekin L: Primary glaucoma in dogs. *J Am Vet Med Assoc* 145:1081–1091, 1964.

20

Surgery of the Skin

The skin is the largest organ of the body, and it is subjected to surgical manipulation to repair traumatic injuries, remove tumors, correct deformities, and treat burns. Skin grafts and pedicle flaps are used routinely in veterinary surgery, which may be as simple as excisional biopsy with a local anesthetic or as complex as transfer of a myocutaneous flap with microvascular anastomosis. It is clear that the level of postoperative concern and possible complications match the procedure itself.

GENERAL POSTOPERATIVE CONCERNS

Hemorrhage

While usually not life-threatening, persistent skin hemorrhage can delay wound healing and create hematomas or seromas. If firm digital pressure fails to stop skin bleeding, the wound may need reexploration and hemostasis.

Self-mutilation

Easy access to many body areas by animals makes self-mutilation an important postoperative complication. Elizabethan collars, bandages, or casts may be needed.

Infection

Given the resident population of skin bacteria and frequent occurrence of contaminated skin wounds, infection of wounds is common. Signs of skin-wound infection include heat, redness, swelling, pain, wound drainage, and unexplained swelling or fluid accumulation. Wound aspiration to collect fluid for analysis and culture is important. Surgical wounds have been classified to provide an estimation of bacterial contamination (Table 20–1). While the guidelines were drawn up for human patients, they also work equally well for dogs and cats.

Many variables influence and contribute to surgical-wound infections. These include preexisting disease, host-defense mechanism, use of immunosuppressive drugs, surgical procedure, method of injury, and both operative and postoperative environment and care. An overall infection rate of 3.5% was found in one report of 4511 patients from a private referral surgical practice (Table 20–2) [1].

Table 20–1
Wound Classification

Clean	Nontraumatic
	No inflammation encountered
	No break in technique
	Respiratory, alimentary, genitourinary tracts not entered
Clean–contaminated	Gastrointestinal or respiratory tracts entered without significant spillage
	Oropharynx entered
	Vagina entered
	Genitourinary tract entered in absence of infected urine
	Biliary tract entered in absence of infected bile
	Minor break in technique
Contaminated	Major break in technique
	Gross spillage from gastrointestinal tract
	Traumatic wound, fresh
	Entrance of genitourinary tract or biliary tract in presence of infected urine or bile
Dirty	Acute bacterial inflammation encountered
	Transection of "clean" tissues for the purpose of surgical access to a collection of pus
	Traumatic wound with retained devitalized tissue, foreign bodies, fecal contamination, and/or delayed treatment

(From Slatter, D.: Textbook of Small Animal Surgery. Philadelphia, W.B. Saunders, 1993. p. 85.)

Skin-Wound Closure

Surgical skin wounds are closed routinely with nonabsorbable sutures or staples, and this technique is termed *primary closure*. Wounds with significant bacterial contamination are closed after 48 to 72 hours. This is termed delayed *primary closure* or *secondary closure*. Table 20–3 summarizes the various techniques of closing wounds.

Pain

Burns, large degloving injuries, and traumatic skin injuries are painful. Appropriate pain control measures should be used.

PLASTIC AND RECONSTRUCTIVE SURGERY

Plastic and reconstructive surgery is now performed with increasing frequency to repair both congenital and acquired defects. Rather than discuss individual procedures, this chapter describes the major types of skin grafts and flaps in use today:

1. Pedicle flaps. The word *flap* denotes a tongue of tissue [2]. Flaps can be classified according to circulation, composition, and location.

2. Subdermal plexus flap. These are pedicle grafts developed without including a direct cutaneous artery or vein.

Table 20–2
Wound Infection Rates Related to Wound Classification in 4511 Patients

Procedure	Number of Cases (% Infected)				
	Clean	Clean–contaminated	Contaminated	Dirty	Overall
Fractures of the pelvis and long bones	1399 (3.5)†	13 (15.4)	9 (22.2)	123 (19.5)	1544 (5.1)
Nonfracture orthopedics: ruptured cruciates, patellar luxations, femoral head ostectomies, dislocated hips and elbows, ostectomies, osteochondroplasties, amputations, pelvic osteotomies, tendon repairs, and total hip replacements	1046 (1.7)	5 (0)	2 (50)	45 (11.1)	1098 (2.2)
Fractures of the mandible/maxilla	11 (0)	24 (4.1)	4 (0)	109 (10.1)	148 (8.1)
Urogenital: castrations, ovariohysterectomies, pyometras, perineal urethrostomies, scrotal urethrostomies, cystotomies, and nephrectomies	146 (0.7)	200 (1.0)	13 (23.1)	23 (8.6)	382 (2.1)
Neurosurgical: hemilaminectomies, laminectomies, spinal fractures, and disc fenestrations	468 (1.1)	0	1 (0)	2 (0)	471 (1.1)
Gastrointestinal: bowel obstructions, gastric volvulus, pyloroplasties, gastropexies, sialoceles, bowel biopsies, and esophageal surgeries	30 (0)	77 (3.8)	10 (1)	8 (0)	125 (3.2)
Miscellaneous: skin tumors, lung lobectomies, anal gland resections, mammary tumors, ear canal ablations and lateral drainages, patent ductus arteriosus, persistent right fourth aortic arch, thyroidectomies, and plastic surgeries	438 (2.1)	107 (0.9)	9 (0)	189 (8.9)	743 (3.6)
Total cases	3538 (2.3)	426 (2.1)	48 (14.6)	499 (11.8)	4511 (3.5)

(From Slatter, D.: Textbook of Small Animal Surgery. Philadelphia, W.B. Saunders, 1993. p. 86.)

3. Axial pattern flap. These are composite flaps that incorporate a direct cutaneous artery and vein (Fig. 20–1). By nature of their blood supply, axial pattern flaps can be used to cover large skin and soft-tissue defects.

4. Composite flap. These are flaps that contain muscle, fat, bone, or cartilage in addition to skin.

5. Split-thickness skin grafts. A skin graft is a segment of epidermis and dermis removed from the body and transferred to a recipient site. Split-thickness grafts contain the epidermis and a variable quantity of dermis. These grafts are indicated in dogs with extensive areas of skin loss; the skin of cats is too thin to allow split-thickness grafts to be harvested [3].

6. Full-thickness grafts. These grafts include the full thickness of the skin.

7. Seed grafts. These are small pieces of skin harvested in an 8- to 10-mm skin trephine and implanted in a recipient bed of granulation tissue. The grafts are suitable for small wounds on the extremities or wounds of uneven contour.

Table 20–3
Summary of Types of Wound Closure/Healing

Primary closure	Clean or clean contaminated wound converted to clean wound	Immediate suture closure of viable tissue without tension
Delayed primary closure	Clean contaminated or contaminated wounds: questionable tissue viability, edema, skin tension	Performed 2 to 5 days after the wound occurs. Lavage and débridement of wound performed while open
Secondary closure	Contaminated or dirty wounds	Performed at least 5 days after injury. Granulation tissue and epithelialized skin edges excised and closure performed
Second intention healing	Wound tissue unsuitable for closure techniques. Large skin defects and extensive tissue devitalization	Healing by granulation tissue, wound contraction, and epithelization

(From Slatter, D.: Textbook of Small Animal Surgery. Philadelphia, W.B. Saunders, 1985. p. 271.)

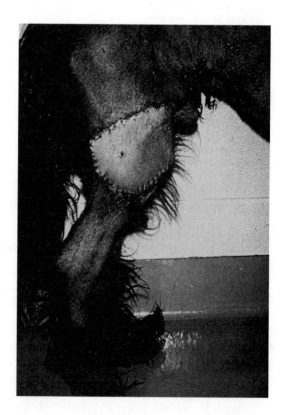

Fig. 20–1. A caudal, superficial, epigastric axial pattern flap used to resurface the medial thigh and stifle following removal of a large hemangiopericytoma. (Courtesy of S.R. Withrow, DVM.)

8. Strip grafts. These are 5-mm wide skin strips placed in a granulation bed. They work well in wounds parallel to the limb axis.

Skin flaps and grafts require diligent postoperative nursing care, including:

1. Drains. Certain grafts (i.e., full-thickness skin grafts) and flaps need some form of continuous wound suction to ensure contact between the graft or flap and the recipient bed. It is important that the drain be secured and continues to operate.

2. Bandaging. The surgical wound should be covered with a sterile, nonadherent bandage and antibiotic ointment (e.g., silver sulfadene), then covered with secondary and tertiary dressing. In some instances, the extremity should be immobilized with a cast or external fixateur to minimize its motion.

REFERENCES

1. Pavletic MM: Pedicle grafts. *In* Slatter D, editor. Textbook of Small Animal Surgery. Philadelphia, 1993, WB Saunders, pp. 295–325.
2. Swaim SF: Skin grafts. *In* Slatter D, editor. Textbook of Small Animal Surgery. Philadelphia, 1993, WB Saunders, pp. 325–340.

21

Surgery of the Endocrine System

THYROID SURGERY

Cats may develop functional tumors of the thyroid, which manifest as hyperthyroidism. The disease is benign in approximately 98% of cases [1] and occurs bilaterally in 70%. Many cats may have hyperthyroid-induced cardiovascular dysfunction. They also may have coexisting diseases such as liver disease, diabetes mellitus, or renal failure. Bilateral thyroidectomy is curative, but it is important to preserve one or more parathyroid glands if possible. Complications of feline thyroidectomy include hemorrhage, damage to the recurrent laryngeal nerve, and hypocalcemic seizures.

In dogs, most thyroid tumors are malignant, and most are nonfunctional (85%) [2]. Surgical removal can be challenging, because the tumors often are locally invasive and possess an excellent and abundant blood supply. Occasionally, they may extend across the midline, necessitating bilateral thyroidectomy. Special postoperative problems include hemorrhage, hypocalcemia (if bilateral thyroidectomy/parathyroidectomy was performed), and surgically related injuries or mortality related to resection of the tumor. It often is difficult to obtain tumor-free margins, thus recurrence is likely.

Hypocalcemia

Serum calcium levels should be measured daily for 3 to 5 days after surgery. If hypocalcemia is detected, clinical signs will develop within 1 to 3 days after surgery. Clinical signs may include restlessness, twitching, muscle tremors, or seizures. If all four parathyroid glands have been removed, calcium supplementation should begin immediately after surgery. To treat acute hypocalcemia, administer a slow intravenous infusion of 1 to 3 ml of 10% calcium gluconate [3], dihydrotachysterol (0.03 mg/kg body weight every 24 hours for 3 days, then 0.01–0.02 mg/kg thereafter), or calcium lactate or carbonate (0.5–3.0 gm orally daily).

Hemorrhage

The surgeon may elect to place a suction drain in the wound bed. The patient should be monitored for hemodynamic instability. Depending on the amount of intraoperative bleeding, an initial packed cell volume/total solids may be needed as a baseline value. Severe hemorrhage left unchecked may produce tracheal pressure and airway compromise.

212

Table 21–1
Drugs Used to Maintain Adequate Blood Glucose Levels in Dogs
with Metastatic Insulinoma

Drug	Dosage	Mechanism
Diazoxide	10 mg/kg/d divided into two doses; can be gradually increased to 30 mg/kg/d	Inhibits beta-cell insulin secretion; raises blood glucose by an extrapancreatic effect
Thiazide diuretics	Chlorothiazine, 20 mg/kg sid/bid; hydrochlorothiazide 2 mg/kg sid/bid	Limits sodium retention and potentiates the action of diazoxide
Propranolol	0.2–1.0 mg/kg tid	Inhibits beta-cell insulin secretion by beta-adrenergic blockade, uncommonly used
Phenytoin	50–80 mg/kg orally tid (in dogs)	Inhibits beta-cell insulin release, uncommonly used and of minimal benefit
Glucocorticoids	0.25–0.50 mg/kg/d divided bid	Promotes gluconeogenesis and peripheral insulin resistance

bid = twice a day; sid = once a day; tid = three times a day.
(From Schear, M, Taboada, J: Metabolic & Endocrine Emergencies. *In* Murtaugh, RJ and Kaplar, DM, Eds. Veterinary Emergency Medicine and Critical Care. St. Louis, CV Mosby, 1992, p. 255.)

Hypocalcemia

If complete thyroidectomy/parathyroidectomy is necessary, alterations in calcium homeostasis may occur, necessitating calcium supplementation (Table 21–1). An initial blood calcium level should be obtained for baseline values, then repeated daily. Supplementation with oral calcium and vitamin D_2 (dehydrotachysterol, 0.02–0.03 mg/kg initially and 0.01–0.02 mg/kg for maintenance) begins with alimentation, and daily calcium level measurements are run for 3 to 5 days. The animal must be observed for signs of hypocalcemia. In addition, thyroid supplementation is necessary.

ADRENALECTOMY

Removal of one or both adrenal glands may be necessary for adrenal cancer or functional hyperplasia. Both an abundant blood supply and the unique location of the adrenal glands make the surgery challenging. Pheochromocytoma is a functional adrenal tumor that produces high levels of catecholamines, which can produce hypertension and tachycardia. These tumors are locally invasive and may extend into adjacent blood vessels. Functional hyperplasia may produce hyperglycemia, electrolyte abnormalities, and slow wound healing. Hemorrhage, wound infection, pneumonia, pulmonary artery thromboembolism, and pancreatitis because of surgical trauma are possible after adrenal surgery. In a study of 25 dogs with adrenocortical neoplasia [4], half of the dogs with adrenocortical carcinoma had metastasis at the time of surgery. Serious complications developed in 50% of cases, with 16 of 25 alive the day after surgery; however of those 16, seven were euthanized at the time of surgery.

A   **B**

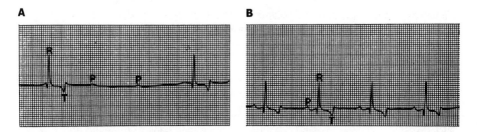

Fig. 21–1. **A,** This electrocardiographic tracing is a lead II rhythm strip from an 8-year-old female mixed-breed dog in addisonian crisis (serum sodium, 122 mEq/L; serum potassium, 8.5 mEq/L). Depicted is complete heart block (more P waves than QRS complexes with no association). **B,** Lead II electrocardiogram from the same dog 3 hours after treatment with desoxycorticosterone acetate, intravenous saline, calcium gluconate, bicarbonate, and insulin-dextrose, illustrating return of normal sinus rhythm. Schaer M: Hypoadrenocorticism. *In* Kirk RW, editor. Current Veterinary Therapy VII—Small Animal Practice. Philadelphia, 1980, WB Saunders, pp. 986–987.

Special concerns include:

1. Pheochromocytoma. If a preoperative diagnosis of pheochromocytoma exists, it is advisable to treat the hypertension and cardiac arrhythmias. Phenoxybenzine hydrochloride (0.2–1.5 mg/kg orally twice daily) is given to lower blood pressure. Propanolol (0.2–2.0 mg/kg orally thrice daily) is used to counteract the arrhythmias. It is important to give the α-blocker phenoxybenzamine before propanolol to prevent propanolol-induced hypertension [5]. The patient's blood pressure must be monitored after surgery, and telemetry is suggested to detect arrhythmias.

2. Hormone supplementation. With bilateral adrenalectomy, glucocorticoids (prednisilone, 0.5 mg/kg twice daily) and mineralocorticoids (Fludrocortisone acetate 0.1 mg/10 kg per body weight per day) are given following surgery. If presurgical abnormalities such as hyperglycemia or hypokalemia exist, they should be monitored following surgery and for 3 to 5 days thereafter.

3. Electrolytes. Thrice daily electrolyte values should be determined. It is important to prevent hypokalemia that might occur with acute adrenal insufficiency. Additional electrocardiographic monitoring may detect evidence of hypokalemia (Fig. 21–1).

INSULINOMAS

Functional tumors of the beta cells in the endocrine pancreas occur in the dog, ferret, and cat. Boxers, German shepherds, and Irish setters [6] have a disposition for the tumor. The insulin-producing tumor causes hypoglycemia because of its secretion of large quantities of insulin (see Table 21–1). Hypoglycemia produces signs referable to central nervous system dysfunction. These include lethargy, weakness, ataxia, tremors, and seizures. Surgery is done to remove tumors from the normal pancreas. Early metastasis is common, and the recurrence rate is nearly 100% [6]. For this reason, surgery is only palliative. In a group of 35 insulinoma patients,

46% had evidence of metastasis at surgery, and the mean survival time for the group was 14.2 months. Diazoxide (10–40 mg/kg orally once daily) was used postoperatively to manage dogs with nonresectable or recurrent insulinomas.

Iatrogenic pancreatitis has been reported in 12 of 29 dogs [7]. In this instance, it is important to continue intravenous fluid therapy and keep the patient NPO for several days.

REFERENCES

1. Salisbury K: Hyperthyroidism in cats. *Compend Cont Ed Pract Vet* 13:1399–1407, 1991.
2. Scavelli TD, Petersen ME: The thyroid. *In* Slatter D, editor. Textbook of Small Animal Surgery. Philadelphia, 1993, WB Saunders, pp. 1514–1523.
3. Schaer M, Taboada J: Metabolic and endocrine emergencies. *In* Murtaugh RJ, Kaplan PM, editors. Veterinary Emergency and Critical Care Medicine. St. Louis, 1992, Mosby–Year Book, pp. 251–272.
4. Scavelli TD, et al: Results of surgical treatment for hyperadrenocorticism caused by adrenocortical neoplasia in the dog: 25 cases. *J Am Vet Med Assoc* 189:1360–1364, 1986.
5. Schaer M, Taboada J: Metabolic and endocrine emergencies. *In* Murtaugh RJ, Kaplan PM, editors. Veterinary Emergency and Critical Care Medicine. St. Louis, 1992, Mosby–Year Book, pp. 251–272.
6. Fingland RB: Surgical diseases of the endocrine pancreas. *In* Slatter D, editor. Textbook of Small Animal Surgery. Philadelphia, 1993, WB Saunders, pp. 1536–1544.
7. Mehlhaff CJ, et al: Insulin producing islet cell neoplasms: surgical considerations and general management in 35 dogs. *JAAHA* 21:607–612, 1985.

APPENDIX

Nutrition in the Hospitalized Patient

CYNTHIA NORDBERG

WHY NUTRITION IS IMPORTANT: HYPERMETABOLISM

The metabolic alterations that occur in starved or fasted normal animals are different from those that occur in starved or fasted *stressed* animals. In simple starvation, metabolic adaptations are made to conserve protein and increase fat usage. Glycogen stores are used up after about 24 hours. Fatty acids are released from fat stores and amino acids are mobilized and used for gluconeogenesis. Fatty acid usage accounts for most of the energy expenditure in healthy starved animals. Protein catabolism provides less than 25% and carbohydrate about 10% of energy needed. Metabolic rate is lowered and energy expenditure is decreased.

The normal metabolic alterations of starvation do not occur in starved ill or injured animals because of the superimposed disease stress. Injury, surgery or illness activates release of TRH and CRH from the hypothalamus, which stimulate release of catecholamines, cortisol, and glucagon. The result is a hypermetabolic state characterized by increased oxygen consumption, catabolism of amino acids from body nitrogen reserves (especially skeletal muscle, plasma proteins, and GI tract) for use in gluconeogenesis, and rapid malnutrition. The consequences of this nutrient depletion include impaired cell-mediated and humoral immunity, decreased resistance to infection, decreased wound strength and wound healing, decreased GI mucosal integrity with subsequent risk of bacterial translocation and sepsis, and eventual progression to multiple organ failure and death.

Early Support Is Important

Nutritional support provides substrates for gluconeogenesis and protein synthesis and provides the energy needed to meet the additional demands of immune system, wound repair, and cell division and growth. Enteral nutrition also helps maintain intestinal mucosal architecture and function.

How Do We Feed?

Feed each patient in a manner as close to physiologically normal as the disease process will allow. Any portion of the GI tract that is functional should be used. ("If the gut works, use it!")

Table A–1

Consequences of Nutrition Depletion

	Starvation	Hypermetabolism
Energy expenditure	↓	↑↑
Mediator activation	↓	↑↑↑
Primary fuels used	Glucose, fat	Glucose, protein, fat
Gluconeogenesis	↑	↑↑↑
Protein synthesis	↓	↓↓
Catabolism	↓ or ↑	↑↑↑
Rate of malnutrition	↑	↑↑↑

Free-choice feeding is best whenever an animal is willing to eat. Free-choice intake can be improved in animals reluctant to eat through good nursing techniques such as hand-feeding, petting and positive reinforcement while the animal is eating, and through improving palatability and aroma by warming the food.

Involuntary feeding can be accomplished by a variety of methods when free-choice intake remains impossible or inadequate. Forced oral feeding via syringe or

Table A–2

Daily Energy Requirements for Hospitalized Patients

Lb	Kg	Cage Rest	Trauma/Surgery/Cancer	Head Trauma/Sepsis/Burns
			Kcal/day	
4	1.8	136	152	206
6	2.7	185	206	280
8	3.6	230	256	347
10	4.5	252	281	381
12	5.4	312	347	470
14	6.4	355	394	535
16	7.3	418	435	590
20	9.1	485	539	732
25	11.4	547	608	825
30	13.6	625	694	942
40	18.2	777	863	1171
50	22.7	917	1019	1383
60	27.3	1053	1170	1588
70	31.8	1181	1312	1780
80	36.4	1307	1452	1970
90	40.9	1427	1585	2151
100	45.4	1543	1714	2326
120	54.5	1769	1966	2668

Table A–3
Undesirable Practices Affecting the Nutritional Status of Hospital Patients

1. Failure to record weight daily or more frequently in acute cases.
2. Rotation of staff at frequent intervals and diffusion of responsibility for patient care.
3. Prolonged administration of glucose and electrolyte solutions without added nutritional support.
4. Failure to observe, measure, and record the amount of food consumed.
5. Withholding food because of multiple diagnostic tests.
6. Failure to recognize and treat increased nutritional needs brought about by injury or illness.
7. Performance of surgical procedures without first making certain that the patient is optimally nourished, and failure to give nutritional support after surgery.
8. Failure to appreciate the role of nutrition in the prevention of and recovery from infection; unwarranted reliance on drugs.
9. Delay of nutritional support until the patient is in an advanced state of depletion which is sometimes irreversible.
10. Limited availability of laboratory tests to assess nutritional status and a failure to use those that are available.

orogastric intubation can be done for short periods (1 to 2 days), but can be frustrating for both the animal and clinician should struggles occur at each feeding.

Drugs such as diazepam, oxazepam, and cyproheptadine may stimulate food intake. However, they are unpredictable and may have significant sedative effects, and intake even with the use of these drugs often remains grossly inadequate.

Nasoesophageal intubation is an excellent option when anesthesia is unavailable or contraindicated. Liquid enteral diets must be used, because most tubes have diameters of only 3.5 to 8 F. Inadvertent tube removal may be a problem in some animals should recurrent sneezing occur or should the patient begin vomiting.

Pharyngostomy/esophagostomy tubes have been used when involuntary feeding must be continued long-term. However, pharyngostomy/esophagostomy tubes are used less often today due to the risk of complications associated with this method of feeding and the widespread use of newer percutaneous techniques for gastrostomy tube placement.

Gastrostomy tubes are an excellent way to provide medium to long-term nutritional support to the patient who is unable or unwilling to take food orally but has a functional GI tract. Tubes are usually well tolerated by animal patients. Blenderized canned foods can be administered through the tube, enabling owners to continue feedings easily at home.

What and How Much Do We Feed?

Water is the nutrient animals require in the largest amount. Water should always be available to patients unless contraindicated. Requirements for normal dogs average 56 to 110 ml/kg/day depending on the size of the dog. Cats require 65 to 80 ml/kg/day. The water requirement in milliliters approximately equals their energy requirement in kcal (to be discussed below).

Energy requirements are affected by many factors, including activity of the animal, specific disease process requiring hospitalization, and acuity of the disease process taking place. To estimate energy needs, begin by calculating basal energy requirement using the following formulas:

$$BER \ = \ 30 \ \times \ Wt(kg) \ + \ 70 \text{ for animals over 2 kg } \quad \text{or}$$
$$70 \ \times \ (Wt(kg))^{0.75}) \text{ for all animals}$$

Then multiply the BER by the "Illness Factor" dictated by the patient's condition to obtain an estimate of the daily illness energy requirement for that patient:

$$
\begin{array}{ll}
\text{Cage rest} & 1.25 \ \times \ BER \\
\text{Surgery/trauma/cancer} & 1.25 \ - \ 1.5 \ \times \ BER \\
\text{Head trauma/sepsis/severe burns} & 1.7 \ - \ 2.0 \ \times \ BER
\end{array}
$$

These numbers are *estimates only;* it is important to assess the patient daily to determine if its energy requirements are being met.

Protein requirements rise markedly during metabolic stress. A negative nitrogen balance occurs quickly in hypermetabolic patients due to increased catabolism. In metabolically stressed humans, protein requirements increase 1.8 to 5 times normal. Current recommendations are to feed high quality protein in quantities to provide for 30 to 48% of total energy requirements in the hypermetabolic patient (4 to 7 grams protein/kg). Disease states such as kidney and liver failure require limited protein intake at 12 to 30% of kcal (2 to 4 grams/kg).

Carbohydrates are a valuable source of energy and glucose, for which there is increased need in hypermetabolism. Unfortunately, many metabolically stressed patients are carbohydrate intolerant and insulin resistant, and they have a limited capacity to oxidize glucose. Foods that are too high in carbohydrates (especially lactose) can cause hyperglycemia and peripheral lactate production. Diarrhea, gas, and abdominal discomfort may also occur due to bacterial fermentation. The current

Table A–4
Percentage of Total Kcal

Product	Protein	Fat	Carbohydrates	Kcal/can
Prescription Diet® Brand Products				
Feline/Canine a/d®	36	50	14	187
Canine p/d®	25	50	25	670
Canine Maintenance®	24	38	38	526
Canine i/d®	25	28	48	559
Canine k/d®	13	49	39	617
Feline p/d®	36	56	7	661
Feline Maintenance®	34	46	20	542 (large can)
Feline k/d®	20	65	14.3	703

Percentages based upon product content of Hill's® Prescription Diet® (Hill's Pet Nutrition, Inc., Topeka, KS) dietary animal food.

Table A–5
The Conditions that Identify Candidates for Nutritional Support

Patients Known to be Protein/Energy Undernourished

Any ICU patient

A history of recent or prolonged weight loss of more than 10% of the body weight

A history of anorexia greater than five days in duration (three days in cases where highly catabolic disease states are suspected)

Generalized loss of muscle mass (chronic protein depletion indicated)

Generalized loss of body fat with loss of skin turgor (chronic energy depletion indicated)

Generalized weakness, lack of appetite, and lethargy for more than five days

Serum albumin concentrations less than the laboratory's minimum low normal range

Total peripheral blood lymphocyte counts of less than $800/\mu l$ when not in severe stress (catecholamine, cortisol axis shifting)

Presence of a nonhealing wound, delayed wound healing, or a decubital ulcer

Presence of a chronic, unrelenting fever or other signs of infection or sepsis

Patients with Conditions Known to Cause Protein/Energy Malnutrition

A post-traumatic state involving severe soft tissue or skeletal injury

Following resection of more than 70% of the small intestine (until adaptation occurs)

Diarrhea caused by severe ulcerative colitis, or any intestinal malabsorption disease state

Severe albumin loss in the urine due to glomerular disease if potentially reversible

Peritonitis, pleuritis, or chylous effusion with effective, progressive drainage

Large open wounds or burns, with persistent exudative losses

Patients with Conditions Associated With Poor Food Intake

Fractures of the mandible or maxilla

Recovering from major oral or nasal surgery

Severe generalized stomatitis, glossitis, pharyngitis, or dental infections

Neurologic conditions such as semicoma, coma, or persistent seizures requiring heavy sedation, tetraplegia, and cranial nerve V and XII palsy

Megaesophagus noted preoperatively or postoperatively, or a disease state associated with it (such as myasthenia gravis)

Extensive gastrointestinal surgery (with prolonged gastric paresis or ileus)

Severe oropharyngeal or cricopharyngeal dysphagia

Esophageal stricture due to a foreign body preventing adequate eating for more than three to five days

Following esophageal surgery (resection)

Following excessive stomach surgery (as with resection) or complicated dilatation torsion

Anorexia with refusal to eat from various medical causes (renal failure, hepatic failure, pancreatitis)

Severe, persistent vomiting or diarrhea

Extensive bowel preps and other forms of workup and treatments that require days of no food intake (e.g. treating pancreatitis)

recommendation for feeding hypermetabolic dogs and cats is for carbohydrates to compose 10% to 30% of the total kcal requirement.

Fat provides a concentrated source of energy. Substituting dietary fat for carbohydrates can reduce or prevent hyperglycemia and increase the energy density of the food. Fat also enhances palatability of the food and improves patient acceptance. Fat should supply 30% to 50% of the total daily kcal requirement for hypermetabolic dogs and cats.

Studies have shown that patients with early enteral nutritional support, administered within hours of injury, have fewer infectious complications, better wound healing, and shorter convalescence than those patients whose nutritional support was delayed. Feeding early has also been shown to suppress the acceleration of metabolic rate by up to 40%.

The clinical goals of nutritional support are to reduce complications, speed recovery, and improve survival. The metabolic goals are to reduce net protein catabolism and to meet nutritional demands of the animal such that body weight is maintained, immune function and wound repair are optimized, and GI integrity and function are maintained.

Who Do We Feed?

Feed all patients that have functional GI tracts! See table A5 for identification of patients especially in need of nutritional support.

REFERENCES

Abood S, Mauterer J, McLoughlin M, Buffington CAT: Nutritional support of hospitalized patients. *In* Slatter (1993). *Principles of Small Animal Surgery.* (W.B. Saunders).

Armstrong Jane: Understanding the metabolic responses to injury and illness in feline and canine patients. *In Enteral Nutrition: Its Importance in Recovery.* (Harmon Smith, Inc., 1992)

Armstrong Jane: Enteral nutrition by tube. *Veterinary Clinics of North America: Small Animal Practice.* 20 (1): 237–271, 1990.

Armstrong Jane: Enteral feeding of critically ill pets: The choices and techniques. *Veterinary Medicine.* September, 1992: 900–909.

Carnevale J, Kallfelz F, Chapman G, Meguid M: Nutritional assessment: guidelines to selecting patients for nutritional support. *The Compendium.* 13 (2): 255–261, 1991.

Chandler M, Greco D, Fettman, M: Hypermetabolism in illness and injury. *The Compendium.* 14 (10): 1284–1290, 1992.

Donoghue Susan: Providing enteral nutritional support for hospitalized patients. *Veterinary Medicine.* September 1992, 910–919.

Donoghue Susan: Nutritional support of hospitalized patients. *Veterinary Clinics of North America: Small Animal Practice.* 19 (3): 475–495, 1989.

Donoghue Susan: Nutritional support of hospitalized animals. *JAVMA.* 200(5): 612–615, 1992.

Kirk C: Nutritional management of metabolic stress. *In Enteral Nutrition: Its Importance in Recovery.* (Harmon Smith, Inc., 1992)

Kronfeld DS: Protein and energy estimates for hospitalized dogs and cats. *Purina International Nutrition Symposium.* January, 1991: 5–11.

Index

Page numbers in *italics* indicate figures; numbers followed by *t* indicate tables.